Creating Consumer Loyalty
in Healthcare

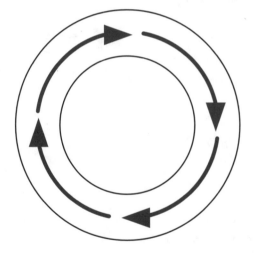

Creating Consumer Loyalty in Healthcare

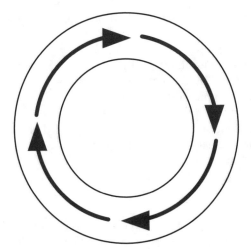

R. Scott MacStravic

Health Administration Press
Chicago, Illinois

03   02   01   00   99   5   4   3   2   1

Library of Congress Cataloging-in-Publication Data

MacStravic, Robin E. Scott.
    Creating consumer loyalty in healthcare / R. Scott MacStravic.
      p. cm. — (ACHE Management Series)
    Includes bibliographical references.
    ISBN 1-56793-108-1 (pbk. : alk. paper)
    1. Patient satisfaction. 2. Customer loyalty. I. Title.
    II. Series: Management series (Chicago, Ill.)
  R727.3.M33   1999
  362.1'068–dc21   99-26390
                                                                         CIP

The paper used in this publication meets the minimum requirements of the American National Standard for Information Sciences—Permanence of Paper for Printed Library Materials, ANSI Z39.48-1984. ∞ ™

Health Administration Press
A division of the Foundation
  of the American College of
  Healthcare Executives
One North Franklin
Suite 1700
Chicago, IL 60606
312/424-2800

Contents

INTRODUCTION

THIS BOOK is about loyalty and about consumers.

It's about loyalty because loyalty has moved from being merely an important value to its current place as the foremost determinant of the success and survival of health plans, healthcare organizations (HCOs), and individual providers. Health plans that can increase their member retention save the costs of replacing lost consumers—often as much as $1,000 per member—even as they enhance their own growth, profitability, and shareholder value. Not only do HCOs and providers that attract and keep their constituencies gain revenue under fee-for-service (FFS) or capitation payment systems, but they improve patient compliance, too, and thus patient outcomes.

And this book is about consumers, because no other single word captures the set of "members" or "enrollees" who apply to health plans, or the "patients," "clients," and "residents" who apply to HCOs and providers. This book does not address other customers, such as employers and government benefit programs, although the importance of their loyalty and the principles of achieving, maintaining, and mining such loyalty have much in common with the principles that apply to consumers.

This book also does not address the conventional approaches to customer loyalty common to other industries. Tricks of the trade when it comes to industrial loyalty, include:

- clubs or other membership organizations that offer special privileges to loyal customers as members;

- frequent flyer, guest, and buyer awards that enable customers to enjoy extra privileges or gain special perks;
- loyalty self-identifiers—special clothing and promotional items with the organization's logo clearly displayed that customers can buy to show their loyalty to a brand or organization;
- smart ID cards—magnetic strip or other information-bearing cards to make it easy for consumers to gain services;
- consumer databases—dossiers and files on individuals and households and their customer behaviors to enable the company to customize communications with them; and
- non-customer communications—ways of keeping in touch with customers between purchases.

All of these tactical approaches are potentially helpful in promoting and sustaining consumer loyalty, but they have been well covered in both standard commercial and healthcare literature. The purpose of this book is to address an entirely different approach to loyalty marketing, one based on a fundamental marketing concept—delivering value to customers and gaining value from them—and on a model called the Loyalty Marketing Wheel.

Delivering Value to Consumers

Although it has long been accepted that the nature of business and the key to marketing is the delivery of value to customers, two distinct notions have developed about the meaning of value in this context. The first idea defines value as quality for the price: essentially everything that is good and helpful about a product or service compared to everything that is bad or harmful about it. This definition positions value within the products or the services themselves, something that organizations or providers own, their banner characteristics as viewed by themselves and by their customers.

The second idea considers value to represent the balance between a benefit and its cost, that is, everything good that happens to customers using a product or service compared to everything bad. Under this definition, value is something owned by the customers; it is *delivered* by organizations but is *gained* by the customers. Where value in terms of quality for price can be the source of admiration and preference among customers, actual benefit for the cost becomes the foundation for loyalty and gratitude. I contend in this book that the benefit-for-cost value stands as the stronger foundation for achieving and maintaining consumer loyalty, and particularly for mining it.

Under the benefit-for-cost definition, value for consumers involves all of the positive versus negative effects of products and services on the quality of consumers' lives. These include both objective—physical—effects and subjective—psychosocial, emotional, and spiritual—effects. These effects are the *outcomes* of the work that health plans, HCOs, and individual providers do to and for the consumer, whereas quality-for-price factors address only their *structures* and *processes*.[1,2]

The structures and processes that health plans, HCOs, and providers manage are the *sources* of the benefit-for-cost outcomes and, therefore, of the value that consumers gain from being customers; however, these sources are not the outcomes and value themselves. The outcomes and value determine how good, how *valuable* the structures and processes are, and thereby how high their quality and price are. But just as outcomes determine the quality and non-monetary price of a service, so, too, do they dictate the benefit-for-cost value that consumers gain.

Although quality-for-price value can involve hundreds, probably thousands of traits of organizations and individuals, benefit-for-cost value involves a limited number of outcomes, products, and services based on what consumers fundamentally value in their lives. A complete delineation of basic consumer *values*, according to various experts, is beyond the scope of this book, but we can summarize them in the following list:

- accomplishment, achievement, making a positive difference
- belonging, social acceptance/respect
- economic well-being
- emotional/mental health
- fun, enjoyment, excitement
- knowledge, skills, wisdom
- physical health
- power, autonomy, freedom
- safety, security, peace
- spiritual health
- self-respect/esteem
- time (discretionary, enough)[3]

(These values may be entirely self-directed, motivating consumers only to the extent that they wish each for themselves—or they may extend to a consumer's family, community, country, or the world as the motivations become increasingly altruistic.)

Delivering value means either protecting or enhancing these fundamental values for consumers. Doing so competitively means delivering more benefit along these value dimensions or less cost, or delivering both compared to the competition. Although health plans, HCOs, and individual providers may measure some of these values in objective terms (for example, physical health, economic health, knowledge/skills, and time), the others are largely subjective values whose perception by consumers is the only measure. And even for objectively measurable effects, the perception of them by the consumer is the key to marketing strategy and therefore to their impact on loyalty.

When the benefit-for-cost impact on consumers is used as the gauge for value delivered, a key dimension of such impact is its *duration*. Many services have only a small, and temporary effect on consumers—making consumers feel respected, welcome, safe, and powerful, for example, during the service encounter itself. The fun and enjoyment of dining at a restaurant or of attending a movie or a play or concert, for example, are unlikely to last long.

By contrast, healthcare has the potential for delivering not only what I call such "during" effects, but also some *enduring* effects. An eye operation may deliver the ability to enjoy movies and the theater for decades to a consumer with serious vision problems. Cosmetic surgery may enhance a consumer's acceptance and respect by others, as well as his or her self-esteem and enjoyment. The medical control of a chronic condition or the cure of an acute problem may enable the consumer to enjoy decades of accomplishment, enjoyment, health, and other values.

In considering both the potential and the reality of delivering value, health plans, HCOs, and providers should consider the duration of the effects they have on consumers, as well as their level of benefit and cost. Because loyalty is a long-term phenomenon, it is likely to be affected as much if not more by the delivery of enduring value as by the effects of the strictly "during" value that last only as long as a particular encounter.

Gaining Value from Consumers

The achievement of consumer loyalty carries with it a number of advantages. Loyal consumers continue to produce capitation revenue so long as they remain loyal, and are more likely to produce fee-for-service revenue as well. By not "defecting," loyal consumers avoid the plan's or the provider's need to replace them just to maintain enrollment or the patient/client/resident base. And loyal customers—typically easier and less expensive to serve—are hence more profitable.[4]

But the real potential in gaining and maintaining loyalty lies not simply in prompting customers' inertia or their consistency as customers. Loyal customers may contribute both through greater quality and quantity as customers, and through their activity in non-customer roles: as self-care providers, advisors, goodwill ambassadors, political allies, volunteers, donors, and in a wide range of roles as highly loyal supporters, as champions of the organization.

Consumer loyalty, by definition, entails the consumer's allegiance to and at least potential for active support and contribution on behalf of an individual or organization.[5] It can entail any number of actions that contribute to the individual's quality of personal or professional life and to the balanced-scorecard performance of the organization.[6] The challenge is first to promote the loyalty of consumers, as the foundation for their making such contributions, and then to devise strategies and tactics that elicit optimal patterns of contributions effectively and efficiently.

Achieving, Maintaining, and "Mining" Loyalty: The Loyalty Marketing Wheel

The related challenges—to achieve, to maintain, and to mine loyalty by delivering value to consumers and gaining value from them—will be addressed in terms of the Loyalty Marketing Wheel. This wheel is formed by two successive value chains.

The Value Delivery Chain

The first chain, which forms the upper half of the wheel, is the value *delivery* chain, a series of steps by which you deliver value to consumers. This is typically the key focus of almost all marketing discussions and activities. The second chain, or the lower half of the wheel, is the value *return* chain, the series of steps by which you can promote the return of consumers' value to you in exchange for the value you have delivered to them.

> **The Five Steps in the Value Delivery Chain are**
> 1. Learning about what consumers value
> 2. Managing the delivery of value
> 3. Promising value to prospective customers
> 4. Tracking the value you deliver to actual customers
> 5. Reminding customers of the value you have delivered

1. Learning about consumer values

This first link in the value delivery chain has two different aims. First is to learn about the values of particular consumers: what they value, what priorities exist among their values. A general understanding of the values of consumers is useful in identifying different segments among them and in developing a familiarity about them that will prove helpful in formulating the strategy aspects of loyalty marketing: deciding which consumers are the best prospects for loyalty marketing and designing the relationship the organization will offer and accordingly deliver.

Second is to learn the particular values that are likely to be crucial in initiating particular transactions with consumers. Offers both of a relationship and of a transaction form the focus of this book. Transactions create the initial introduction of consumers to the organization and act as the source of most instances of value delivery. Based as they are on exchanged value, transactions are the key foundation for loyalty marketing. Without accurate knowledge of the right values to work on, the management, promises, tracking, and reminders to consumers of value delivered will work only by chance.

2. Managing value delivery

Always a personal frustration of mine has been the fact that while marketing often has almost total control over the *learning* process regarding consumer value, it has almost no control over the actual delivery of the value. This is the responsibility of management in healthcare and other service industries (and of manufacturing in the durable goods industries). Even though marketing can conjure up irresistible offers based on what it learns about the values important to consumers, management gets to decide, arrange for, and direct the delivery of the value that consumers get.

When significant discrepancies appear between the offer that market research calls for and what management comes up with as the offer is actually delivered, a number of bad things can result. The worst is that the offered product or service—as it is delivered—will not match what consumers want. This will undermine all attempts to attract consumers to the offer, and it will undercut even the potential for consumer satisfaction—not to mention loyalty.

When marketers get back into the act in their marketing communications, they may promise value to consumers in order to attract them; the consumer will be led to expect value that management ends up not delivering. This will promote consumer dissatisfaction and defection, and it will generally hamper the achievement and maintenance of consumer loyalty.

Without a good fit between learning and management, management may overdo the delivery of value in the sense of delivering benefits at too high a cost to the organization. This may drive the price of the offer past its competitive edge, and may thereby prevent the achievement of the transactions that can initiate and reinforce loyalty. It can also drive the return on investment for loyalty marketing efforts into the red, either preventing their implementation if poor returns are estimated in advance or eliminating the effort if those poor returns are discovered after the fact.

On the other hand, if the best offer imagined is not turned into reality by management in some way, nothing will happen. I'm not sure that marketers would be more successful than managers at designing, arranging, and day-to-day delivery responsibilities, or that they'd even be willing to take them on. The key to successful loyalty marketing, indeed to successful transaction marketing in general, is to achieve the best possible fit among learning, management, and communication.

3. Promising value

Making a value promise actually belongs in the middle of the management sequence. Management normally designs and arranges for the delivery of value before promising it to prospects. But with services, unlike goods, the promises must precede delivery and must succeed in attracting customers before delivery can occur. (The three management challenges were presented together, before the communications challenges, because they are so closely connected and not because they all belong there in the time sequence.)

Your aim in "promising" value is directed to creating confidence in the minds of consumer prospects that they can expect to get the value they want—and that you intend to deliver it. This does not actually mean to "promise" value. However, you do want prospects to feel assured of receiving the value you describe, so it is often best to think of your communications as promises. You may win over prospects if they see unique or superior value in your offer, or you may create higher confidence in their minds that they will actually get the desired value from you (compared to some doubts about your rivals), or both.[7]

4. Tracking value delivered

Tracking value, that is, measuring the value that has actually been delivered, and particularly the degree to which that value has been perceived by consumers, is a step often given short shrift by healthcare providers and plans. They may check to see if the objective outcomes they were after for their own quality measurement, such as clinical parameters for medical quality and consumer satisfaction scores for service quality, have been acheived. But rarely do they measure the impact of their individual consumer encounters or relationships on that consumer's quality of life.

Without tracking, you cannot be sure that you are delivering any value, or are doing so effectively and efficiently. Tracking can identify dissatisfied consumers and their reasons for dissatisfaction before you start to see defections, that is, early enough for your recovery from failures and your ability to win consumers back. Moreover, tracking, by producing data and identifying delighted consumers, can be used in making your promises about value more effective. And tracking provides the basis for the next step in the value delivery chain.

5. Reminding consumers of value delivered

This last step in the value delivery chain is the one least prevalent in health plan and provider communications. Such marketing communications focus almost exclusively on the predicting and promising role of communications as they endeavor to win new consumers rather than merely to keep the ones they have. And although promise/prediction communications can rely on mass media and usually do, efforts at reminding should be customized to individuals—and more so than is typically included in what we call mass customization.[8]

Reminders can include reports to consumers on value effects (or at least on outcomes that connect with value effects) that you track in your own records. It can also include value effects that you get consumers to keep track of themselves, since their tracking reminds them of value delivered every time they record it for themselves. Reminders can also include your surveys and individual follow-up interviews of consumers to check on their perceptions of value, because asking them about value also serves as a reminder to them as they answer.

The value you track and remind consumers of may involve the results of a single encounter, an episode of care, a continuing relationship, or any mix of the three. The more that value is delivered specifically through a relationship, and the more that value is of the enduring versus the "during" variety, the more likely it is that value will promote loyalty in contrast to mere satisfaction.

In addition to reminding consumers about the value they have gained, you may choose to remind your own internal stakeholders about the value you have delivered. This reminder may occur via annual reports to shareholders, regular bulletins to your employees and physicians, or other communications devices. You may also report the value you have delivered to the community, your volunteers, and donors: the positive difference you have made to the quality of life of the community (in contrast to the tax exemption–protecting reports of the efforts and expenditures you have made). The intent is to enable these stakeholders to feel proud of what you have done and to support rather than hinder you in your overall efforts.

You may also translate the quality of life value you have delivered to consumers into performance value delivered to other customers. If a provider achieves better outcomes in a shorter time for patients, that may translate into lower costs for health plans and higher member satisfaction.

The success of a health plan or a provider in enabling consumers to manage their own symptoms or chronic conditions can translate into lower absenteeism, improved productivity, and lower operating costs for employers. Reminding those customers, as well as consumers, of value delivered should help in both attracting and retaining those customers.

Once you have implemented the five steps of the value delivery chain, you should be able to identify the value you have delivered and the extent to which consumers are aware of it, appreciate it, and give you credit for it. You can evaluate the results of your work up to now, at this point, in terms of consumer loyalty, using measures of loyalty reflecting their attitudes toward you. You could stop here, as a matter of fact, and leave to billing and collections any questions of the consumers returning value to you. You could start the value delivery chain over again at this step, to get consumers to be better customers.

You could focus your attention on improving (or at least maintaining) your present value delivery performance to retain a greater number of consumer patients and members. In cases where just keeping consumers as customers has a high intrinsic value, this may be as far as you wish to go—perhaps keeping the patients and enrollees for their present and future pmpm payment contributions alone. You could aim no higher than seeing to it that your present patients pay their bills more promptly or with less effort and cost to you. Or you could hope that more satisfied and loyal consumers could add even greater value to your efforts by becoming "better" customers.

As a FFS–paid provider, you could aim, for example, for a higher frequency of the present value transactions you are having with consumers (i.e., frequency marketing). As a health plan or provider at risk, on the other hand, you could aim for a *lower* frequency of such transactions. You could plan to initiate new types of transactions that consumers have not engaged in before, such as buying other forms of insurance or other services from you (cross-marketing), and, to some degree, you could steer consumers to higher-priced or more profitable transactions (up-marketing). Or, if you're at risk, you could concentrate on lower-priced transaction options (down-marketing) or nonuse of services (de-marketing).[9]

If you think you are already getting as much as you can in *customer* value return from your consumers, or if you see great potential from other contribution roles as well, your objective may be to gain added value from consumers via any of the other roles they might play, from self-care to collaboration to volunteering, advising, donating, governing, word-of-mouth advertising, and so on. However broad or narrow, conventional or innovative your ambitions, you should next consider the value return chain.

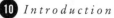

The Value Return Chain

This chain also consists of five steps, similar to the value delivery steps, that you can take to initiate, maintain, and increase the value your consumers return to you.

The Five Steps in the Value Return Chain
6. Evaluating consumer loyalty
7. Promoting consumers' returning value to you
8. Monitoring the value you gain in return
9. Acknowledging the value you have gained
10. Sharing the value returned with its contributors

6. Evaluating consumer loyalty

Once you have reached the end of the value delivery chain, it is a good time to evaluate your organization's effect, so far, on consumer loyalty. This means not only evaluating the status and value of loyalty as the intended outcome, but assessing the value contributed by each of the separate steps in the value delivery chain. How much effect have the learning, managing, promising, tracking, and reminding steps had, individually and collectively, on the differences you have made in consumers' levels of loyalty?

The second challenge in the loyalty evaluation step lies in assessing the extent to which particular consumers are good prospects for returning value to you. You need to evaluate both their general predisposition to return value to you and their attitudes toward the specific contributions you have in mind. This requires, of course, that you have clear ideas on their probable contributions, as well as an active vision of the kinds of value you would like them to return.

If you are new to the idea of soliciting contributions of value from your consumers (beyond asking them to pay their bills on time), you can look into the performance problems and aspirations with which they can help you and the roles you think are possible for them to assume. Published descriptions of the contributions of loyal consumers to the plans and providers they've admired should give you new ideas on specific contributions you might elicit. You can brainstorm possibilities with your staff or with consultants; you can also treat the potential for consumer participation as a challenge to be addressed *jointly* by you and the consumers.

If your consumers are at least somewhat loyal or favorably disposed toward you—if they are mildly interested in your success and survival for any reason—they may be willing to sit down beside you and work on determining possibilities. Your consumers may help you both address those possibilities and discover why these persons are not making particular contributions now, or the missing factor that would make the idea of particular contributions more appealing.

7. Promoting value return contributions

Encouraging and enabling loyal consumers to contribute value to you is, for the most part, a marketing challenge. Because value contributions involve consumers rather than employees or even staff physicians, this is obviously a marketing function, and management should recognize it as such.[10] Prompting consumer participation involves communicating with them, mainly, even if only to ask them for a particular effort or contribution or to otherwise make them aware of what you would like them to do. This normally increases the probability and frequency of a return of value by consumers far beyond the results you realize through mere wishful thinking about the "return of a favor."

All of the forms of communication used in step 2 to promote consumer acceptance of your value offer are applicable to prompting their return of value. In practice, however, more personalized communications methods tend to work better and to reinforce your relationship with loyal consumers as well. The great thing about consumer contributions that return value is that those contributions also tend to promote and reinforce consumer loyalty as well as added value to your performance.[11]

Most industries—certainly most health organizations—seek an extremely limited scope of value return. Consumers and third parties responsible for their bills are expected to pay for the services they have received; moreover, such payment is expected whether or not a desired amount of value has been delivered. Healthcare providers charge for *effort*, not results, that is, for the structures they maintain and the processes they manage, rather than for the outcomes they achieve or the value consumers gain.

This is perhaps reflected best in the fact that providers charge high fees even when patients die in the Emergency Room. When a patient found without a heartbeat and artificially resuscitated is subjected to unsuccessful CPR and other life support services and never regains consciousness—that is, when treatment makes no difference—the family is still charged for the effort expended. I am not suggesting that this time-honored practice be abandoned, but it does hinder loyalty marketing if you expect returned value and none has been delivered.

Moreover, when the aim is to get payment in return for value delivered, to whom do we give the responsibility for billing and collections? The finance function! Although this may make sense from a management perspective, it is likely to be suboptimal at best and, at worst, in direct conflict with loyalty marketing. Hospital bills tend to be a mystery to most consumers, and the billing/collection process, annoying at best, is maddening in many cases. Rarely do finance functions put consumer satisfaction and loyalty high on their list of performance criteria and rarely are they the basis for manager and staff bonuses.

Promoting returned value can be as important a marketing challenge as promoting the acceptance by consumers of your initial value transaction offer. Its worth clearly will vary depending on the amount of value you can gain in return, but this can become a chicken-or-egg dilemma. Do you plan and budget your return value effort based on the value that consumers have already returned—which may be too little to finance a successful effort—or do you plan and implement your effort and then see what it produces in returned value?

8. Monitoring returned value

The reasons for monitoring the value you gain from consumers are essentially the same as those for tracking the value you deliver. Tracking tells you and organizational reviewers your level of success, and it lets you modify particular efforts as needed. It can also help strengthen your promotion efforts if your successes in eliciting value return contributions are tracked and then recognized or rewarded. And monitoring provides the basis both for reminding people about the value they gain (step 9) and for sharing the value you gain (step 10).

Unlike tracking the value you've delivered, where your own records are limited as a source of useful measures, monitoring the value consumers have returned relies mainly on your own records. Some contributions will not appear in your records, however, such as how loyal consumers have been, given a choice—whether they have resisted approaches by your rivals. You will have to rely on surveys and other means of obtaining self-reported information for these kinds of contributions of value. To learn how many of your loyal consumers have referred their friends, for example, you have to ask new patients or enrollees if they were referred and, if so, by whom, so that you can both track this kind of returned value and thank loyal referrers for their effort.

9. Acknowledging returned value

Acknowledging the value that consumers have contributed is first a means of publicizing and relating the importance of their contributions to you, showing them you have made the effort both to track and to report their contributions. Acknowledgment also helps to reinforce the effect of contributions on strengthening loyalty, because consumers will be aware of their contributions first when they make them and again when they are told about them. And reminding internal stakeholders about the value consumers have contributed should add to stakeholder appreciation of the importance of consumers, and from there to support for future consumer loyalty efforts and investments.

Because your own records are the primary source for information about consumer contributions, you typically have to report them to the consumers yourself, rather than to rely on them to track their own contributions. You also need to translate the contribution, which is all they know, into its actual value to you—just as you translate your records of clinical outcome data for consumers to make them knowledgeable about what delivered value means.

10. Sharing the value contributed

To suggest that you share the value you have gained with the consumers who contributed it may seem revolutionary and perhaps ridiculous to many readers. It is simply, however, a logical application of our understanding of successful and lasting relationships. In most cases, relationships work when both parties see them as fair and equitable and because they involve not only win-win effects on both parties, but WIN-WIN, rather than WIN-win effects.[12] Sharing the value returned is the most direct approach to promoting perceptions of fairness among those consumers who have contributed value.

Sharing does not mean splitting every dollar of return value, with each party getting half. It simply means determining and implementing methods of sharing that both parties consider to be fair and that reinforce (or at least do not undermine) the loyalty relationship. Consumers may be satisfied when you invest in community benefit initiatives, rather than devoting all of the value you gained from them to increasing shareholder dividends and executive compensation, for example. They may be delighted if you donate a portion of your gains to a charity or community effort they support.

As you learn about consumer loyalty in preparation for prompting their return contributions, you may discover that many are so grateful for your value delivered that they will be delighted to "give back," asking no type of sharing in return. In my experience, consumers have been conservative in suggesting the best ways to share the value they have contributed. On the other hand, if they demand outrageous "compensation" in return for their contributions, making your return on your loyalty investment a loss proposition, you surely have a right to forget the whole thing, or at least to negotiate a mutually acceptable alternative.

Completing the Wheel

The value return chain almost completes the Loyalty Marketing Wheel; at least it forms the lower half of the wheel in the illustration. The only step missing is to work the wheel in continuous revolutions. Your loyalty marketing effort cannot end with one rotation; the process requires continuous repetition through all of the steps of both chains. Moreover, it requires that you think and behave as loyally to consumers as you wish them to do on your behalf. In most cases, you have to show the way, demonstrating what Bell calls "abundance" as a prerequisite to success in relationship development. The party who initiates the relationship effort must be willing to invest up front with no certainty of an acceptable return, to make the first move, and to accept less than might be considered a fair exchange rather than insisting on no risks.[13]

You must be willing to commit to promoting loyalty before you can be sure you will gain from it. Unless you first invest in promoting loyalty by promising and delivering value (preferably including tracking and reminding consumers about the value you have delivered as well), and then in promoting, tracking, reminding, and sharing the value of return contributions, you cannot know your consumers' potential for loyalty. You can start on a trial basis, of course, to see if it seems a worthy investment, by selecting a small sample of consumers for your value marketing program and monitoring the value you gain in return.

The ten steps in developing the Loyalty Marketing Wheel will certainly include some ideas (perhaps many) that you have never tried before. In discussions with healthcare providers and health plans around the country, I have found *no one* who practices all of the ten steps (although there may be some that I simply have not run across). Variations are great in terms of the persons and organizations tracking value delivered—and including it in performance assessments and bonus arrangements, for example—and in the ways in which those providers and plans are doing so.

Formal and comprehensive reminder systems of value delivered to consumers are virtually nonexistent as far as I can tell—I found only one example of a physician sending an annual health status improvement report to his patients.[14] Organizations that employ health risk assessments send annual reports to individual consumers on their health status and risk changes, summarizing the value of such changes in terms of gains or losses in life expectancy.[15] And reports on performance value delivered to employers have sometimes been sent by plans[16] and providers.[17]

But if this means that I cannot point to successful implementers of the Loyalty Marketing Wheel as benchmark organizations to follow, it also means that this model offers opportunities to make quantum leaps, as opposed to modest increments, in loyalty marketing success. If you and your rivals have gone no further than step 3 or 4 in the value delivery chain, and you can plan and implement the other six or seven, you stand to gain far more of an advantage than you would using a purely incremental approach. You could become known as *the* innovator in your market for as many as six or seven new ways of increasing, maintaining, and "mining" consumer loyalty; you could even be the first to initiate a loyalty effort of any kind.

About This Book

Part I describes the top half of the Loyalty Marketing Wheel as it stands in place linking the five steps for *delivering* value to consumers (see Figure 1 on page 16). This first half addresses loyalty-focused approaches to learning about consumers, selecting loyalty prospects, designing a loyalty offer, and delivering that offer. The communication of that offer, the act of promising value to prospective loyal consumers, comes next followed by the tracking of delivery efforts to see what value has actually been delivered to consumers and perceived by them as value. A novel step in marketing communications comes next: the reminders to consumers about value they have gained, in your own explicit pursuit of high levels of loyalty.

Part II covers the second (lower) half of the Loyalty Marketing Wheel, securing return-value contributions from consumers. It begins with addressing ways to evaluate the success of value delivery in achieving consumer loyalty and the predisposition of customer-consumers to make return contributions. Particulars of promoting specific contributions are then covered, together with discussions of methods to use in tracking the contributions and their value to the organization—and of ways to remind consumers and others of what they have contributed. The book ends by discussing an idea that belongs particularly to the loyalty of consumers and their contributions of value: that of sharing the value contributed with those who made the contributions.

Although the literature and experience of dealing with consumer loyalty cover much more ground than I can include in this book, my intent is to motivate readers and to enable them to learn the essential concepts and to identify at least the essential steps for achieving, maintaining, and "mining" consumer loyalty in healthcare. The investment required to bring about significant levels of consumer loyalty and to realize the potential of return-value contributions will be major; loyalty marketing is no simple minor modification to current transaction marketing. But

Figure 1   The Loyalty Marketing Wheel

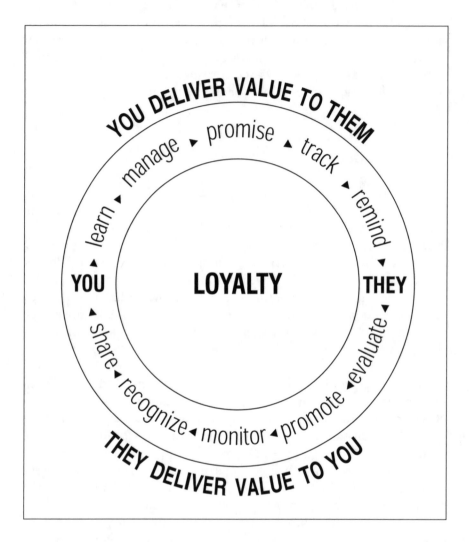

the return on that investment can include a greater impact on your organization and on consumers than you have ever imagined.

References

1. Donabedian, A. 1966. "Evaluating the Quality of Medical Care." *Milbank Memorial Fund Quarterly* 44: 166–203.
2. ———. 1980. *The Definition of Quality and Approaches to its Assessment.* Chicago: Health Administration Press.

3. MacStravic, S., and G. Montrose. 1998. "Behavioral Foundations." In *Managing Health Care Demand,* pp. 97–118. Gaithersburg, MD: Aspen.

4. Reichheld, F. 1993. "Loyalty-Based Management." *Harvard Business Review* 71, no. 2 (March/April): 64–73.

5. *Merriam-Webster's Collegiate Dictionary, 10th ed.,* 1998. 691. Springfield, MA: Merriam-Webster.

6. Kaplan, R., and D. Norton. 1996. *The Balanced Scorecard: Translating Strategy into Action.* Boston: Harvard Business School.

7. MacStravic, S. 1998. "Marketing by Means of the Confidence Factor." *Health Care Strategic Management* 16, no. 1 (January): 1, 19–23.

8. Adamson, G. 1998. "In Your Face." *Managed Healthcare* 8, no. 4 (April): 15–16, 21–22.

9. Kotler, P., and R. Clarke. 1987. *Marketing for Health Care Organizations,* p. 16. Englewood Cliffs, NJ: Prentice-Hall.

10. MacStravic, S. 1997. " 'Managing' Demand: The Wrong Paradigm." *Managed Care Quarterly* 5, no. 4 (autumn): 8–17.

11. Fisk, T., C. Brown, K. Cannizzaro, and B. Naftal. 1990. "Creating Patient Satisfaction and Loyalty." *Journal of Health Care Marketing* 10, no. 2 (June): 5–15.

12. Srinivasan, M. 1996. "When It Comes To Loyal Customers, The I's Have It." *Marketing News* 30, no. 14 (1 July): 4.

13. Bell, C. 1994. *Customers as Partners: Building Relationships That Last.* San Francisco: Berrett-Koehler.

14. Baker, S. 1998. *Managing Patient Expectations,* p. 251. San Francisco: Jossey-Bass.

15. Personal Wellness Profile®. Wellsource, Inc., Clackamas, OR.

16. Goedert, J. 1998. "Tufts Puts Its Data to Good Use." *Health Data Management* 6, no. 7 (July): 44–46.

17. "The Cleveland Clinic Foundation: A Commitment to Strong Relationships." *Healthcare Strategy Alert* (January 1998): 7–8.

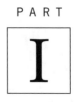
The Value Delivery Chain

Introduction to Part I

Part I covers the first (top) half of the Loyalty Marketing Wheel, the delivery and demonstration of value to achieve consumer loyalty. It begins with the first chapter, "Learning About Loyalty," in which five categories of information needed in the pursuit of loyalty are noted together with the ways in which each affects subsequent steps in value delivery. It offers an overview of some recommended information techniques uniquely suited to loyalty marketing.

Chapter 2, "Managing Value Delivery," discusses the roles of management in delivering value to the consumer loyalty prospects identified in the first, learning step. Challenges to meet in designing the loyalty offer are then discussed along with particular transaction offers, leading to a description of management's development of specific value offers to deliver. The final discussion in this chapter examines the significant ongoing challenges that management encounters in delivering the intended—and most effective and efficient—value package.

Chapter 3, "Promising Value," presents the communications step. The organization "promises" value to consumers at this point, in an effort to attract them to the transactions that create the beginning of a loyal relationship. Factors that guide decisions on the value to promise are described together with the risks and advantages of each. Some suggestions are offered on ways to promise value, recognizing the special risks as well as the advantages involved in promising outcomes and value in healthcare.

Chapter 4, "Tracking Value Delivered," addresses the next step: learning the kinds and amounts of value that have been delivered to and actually perceived by the consumer. Most organizations settle for tracking the satisfaction of customers, plus the revenue or other gains the organization realizes from delivering value; however, loyalty marketing advances greatly if the nature of value delivered to consumers is tracked along with the two usual measures. This tracking serves both to reinforce and improve the management task of delivering value, while it begins the process and provides the foundation for the next step, providing reminders to consumers. The chapter discusses recommended tracking methods and the key uses of tracking in loyalty marketing.

Chapter 5, "Reminding Consumers of Value Delivered," completes the discussion of the value delivery chain by describing the novel and rarely practiced idea of reminding consumers that the value you promised has indeed been delivered. This step completes the loop begun in the third chapter by adding to consumers' awareness and appreciation of value delivered, and their attribution of that value to the efforts of the plan or provider responsible for it, thus promoting loyalty far better, certainly, than silence could. The chapter ends with some recommended approaches to reminding.

LEARNING ABOUT LOYALTY

Figure 1-1

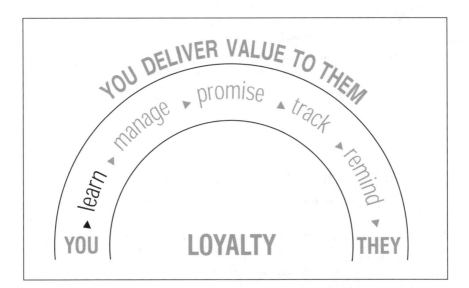

YOU DELIVER VALUE TO THEM

learn ▸ manage ▸ promise ▸ track ▸ remind

YOU   LOYALTY   THEY

LEARNING ABOUT loyalty differs substantially from conventional marketing research, which focuses on transactions. In the first place, *the subject* to be learned is different, emphasizing perceptions and attitudes about relationships, not just about encounters, and about *durable value,* not merely the "during" value mentioned in the

Introduction. And in the second place, the purpose of the techniques you use in learning about foundations for loyalty is both to promote any existing loyalty and to take advantage of it while you are learning.

Learning the Consumer

Learning about customers is at the heart of the marketing paradigm, and is at least as important to loyalty marketing as to transactions. For that reason, this is the longest chapter in the book, reflecting both the vital contribution that learning makes and the complexity of the challenge. It addresses, in five categories, the kinds of things worth learning about consumers in pursuing their loyalty as well as the methods to use in learning (the latter only briefly, in the special context of loyalty marketing):

1. information on the *potential value to you* of consumer loyalty, advantages available through the loyalty of particular consumers, and which of those advantages hold the most potential value for you;

2. information on the *probability* of loyalty, how likely it is that loyalty can be achieved with particular consumers and who the most likely prospects are;

3. information on what *particular consumers* are looking for as *reasons for wanting* a relationship with a plan or provider;

4. intelligence that will be useful in pursuing loyalty among *particular populations of consumers*; and

5. information on the *current status of loyalty* among consumers of interest.

1. The Potential for Value in Consumer Loyalty

The potential of consumers to become your customers—the beginning of a loyalty marketing process—is both a function of the consumers and of your organization. What are these people looking for; what values motivate them in general; what causes them to choose one hospital, nursing home, primary physician, specialist, traditional health insurer, or HMO over another? What does your organization offer that connects with these values and selection criteria; that is, what unique or superior benefits can you deliver compared to the benefits of rival organizations?

What is the likelihood that a particular consumer (or group of consumers) will be a good customer, one you want to attract and retain? Being a "good" customer can mean using plenty of your services, if you are paid on a fee-for-service (FFS) basis—or as few as possible if you're paid on the basis of capitation and sharing risk. In many cases, paying promptly and completely is also part of being a good customer. "Good" can also mean using the right services at the right time and in the right setting to help you improve your quality and efficiency, or conscientiously taking advantage of all of the appropriate preventive and early detection services that will enable you to provide quality, health impact, and long-range cost control. To sum up, most marketing efforts have dual goals: to attract and retain the best as well as the most customers possible.

The history of consumers' behavior as customers is some of the most valuable information you can collect. Finding out which consumers have been "high users" of health services in the past or, in general, which types of people tend to be high users, can help FFS providers identify the most promising prospects and can help both health plans and at-risk providers determine those of whom to be wary; on the other hand, if payment systems are based on health status and risks, the most desirable consumers for providers and plans at risk can be chronic disease patients.[1] The highest users, that is, the 30 percent of consumers responsible for 75 percent of healthcare expenditures, are of greatest interest either way.[2]

Determining which consumers have been the most profitable, or are likely to be, is a standard approach for selecting loyalty prospects. Checking which of them have been too much trouble or too expensive to serve, or too demanding or difficult for staff to deal with, for example, can help in screening out weak marketing prospects.[3] A "customer portfolio analysis" can at least identify "who has been how valuable" to your organization in the past and can help predict the consumers who will probably hold the most future value.[4]

Obtaining information on households, as opposed to individuals by themselves, is a potentially helpful tactic in pursuing consumer loyalty.[5] A household, or even an extended family living in the same market, can be affected by the same value delivery efforts, enjoy the same benefits, or at least appreciate those benefits. Obtaining information from members about a household is usually more efficient than focusing on one person at a time. And when, later in the loyalty marketing process, we remind consumers of value delivered, and we promote and track return contributions, the process is likely to be more efficient on a household basis.

To make the best selections of prospects for consumer loyalty, it is necessary to gain insight into which of them have the greatest potential for *all* contribution categories—not merely for the customer role. The history of particular prospects, or of people like them as reported in published research, can suggest those consumers who have made particular contributions; generally speaking, such consumers are more likely than others to make similar future contributions.

Put simply, the potential of individual consumers or particular consumer groups can be expressed as their lifetime dollar value to you: the amounts they may contribute to your bottom line each year times the number of years they may be loyal or at least retained as customers. This is based on the expected fee-for-service revenue or capitation premiums each might yield, minus the costs of serving them. Because their revenue impact and your costs of serving them are subject both to unpredictable change and your own management efforts, such predictions will necessarily be estimates.

Moreover, you will find their potential value to increase as you learn how to "mine" the loyalty potential of consumers more effectively, expanding the number of roles they play relative to your organization and the scope of your performance values that they affect. And as you learn increasingly to reinforce and maintain their loyalty, and to elicit particular contributions of value from them, your probability of realizing that potential will increase. After reading this book, you should find that your original estimates of the value of consumers were quite conservative.

2. The Probability of Attracting and Keeping Loyal Consumers

The ideal would be to estimate (and even calculate) the potential value of particular consumers in dollar terms. To select the ones to attract, however, you would want to multiply that potential value times the probability of getting them to be loyal, to fulfill their potential, with the product allowing you to rank-order the best prospects for loyalty initiatives. Even if you cannot reach a reliable and meaningful estimate of potential dollar value, however, it is helpful to estimate probability.

Identifying your best loyalty prospects can begin with determining those who have gained the most value, and particularly those who already perceive the value you have delivered to them in the past, highly appreciate that value, and attribute most or all of it to your efforts and not to other causes. Learning which consumers anticipate future contact with you and look forward to value from you is equally useful in identifying the most probable loyalists.

How satisfied are they with past encounters? Even though satisfaction is only partially correlated with loyalty, high levels of your measures of satisfaction are good predictors of likely loyalists. How do they rate you as a "quality" provider or plan, in prestige and reputation, compared to your rivals?[6] Even if they have not had any experience with you, if they rate you high and rank you at or near the top, your chance of gaining their loyalty is comparatively better.[7]

How do they rate you in terms of being a "good value for the money"? My own research has indicated that such value ratings by patients are most closely linked to their stated intentions to return to the hospital where they were treated and to recommend it to others. It also indicates that, on average, they consider a hospital to be a very poor value, highly overpriced, even given the great and durable benefits their stay has gained for them. The practice of listing hospital prices on patient bills, even where the actual payments received will be significantly lower, surely tends to promote this poor perception of value.

What are consumers' values, goals, aspirations, and problems? In what ways do their values align with those of your organization? Do they want the services you can deliver—and deliver better than your rivals? Do they see value in loyal relationships, in general, and particularly with your organization?[8] Do they have the personality[9] or belong to the demographic (e.g., seniors) or psychographic segments known to be more prone to loyalty or not interested in it?[10] Do they want the kind of relationship you are interested in? (For instance, if you are a physician, do they want you as an authority, a partner, or a coach?)[11]

If you are a health plan, is their primary provider in your network, or would they have to change doctors if they enrolled? And how loyal are they to their physician? How do they rate your member services, known to be a high predictor of overall satisfaction and reenrollment?[12] Did they choose you, or were they offered only one plan choice? (Those who have no choice are less likely to be loyal.)[13] Do they indicate a specific intention to reenroll or defect? While such intentions are less than perfect predictors of actual behavior, they can suggest good and bad prospects, and warn you of those at risk for defection.[14]

How do consumers feel about you in particular? Do they perceive that you understand their concerns?[7] Are they thinking about other providers? Does their interest in a different one show a clear intention to switch? What levels of trust, familiarity, interdependence, interest in your success and survival, sense of shared values, and other relationship-promoting perceptions do they now have?[15] How do they rate you overall as a relationship prospect, both in absolute terms and relative to their other known options?

Their responses to past relationship problems with health plans and providers can offer insights into their possible behavior toward you. Have they tended to defect at the first service failure or bad experience? Have they voiced their concerns and given you and other organizations a chance to recover and thereby to keep them as customers? Have they simply hung on in silence waiting for another option, or have they maintained strong loyalty in spite of occasional failures?[16] Such information can help you assess not only their probable loyalty, but their value to you as well.

Learning the consumers who have made particular contributions in the past also provides both types of insights. People who have contributed to your efforts are more likely to make a repeat contribution than are noncontributors to do so the first time. They are also more likely to make contributions in other categories if they have already made them in one; for example, volunteers are more likely to donate than are nonvolunteers.[17] If your research detects the kinds of people who are more likely to make particular kinds of contributions (e.g., retired people more likely to volunteer), you can use that information in your efforts to attract loyalty.

3. The Expectations and Wishes of Consumers

What do consumers see as likely benefits of a loyal relationship with a hospital, physician, or plan, and which of those benefits do they want? Because relationships are two-sided, consumers are likely to go through a process much like yours in selecting loyalty prospects. Which particular benefits do they see as available from you—and about which are they not so sure? What overall benefits do they see from experiencing a loyal relationship with you as opposed to having only occasional encounters?[18] In what ways do consumers wish their quality of life to be protected or enhanced by dealing with you or anyone like you?[19]

What are the benefits to them in the characteristics about you that have influenced their past and present loyalty levels?[20] By pinpointing the factors that have determined current customers' past satisfaction with your organization and their present loyalty to it, you can learn what will make a difference to them in the future. By learning the reasons behind any contributions they have made to other organizations, you can gain new insights into prospects of your own.

What specific kinds of help do consumers hope for from you if they are current customers, or from organizations such as yours if they're prospects? One study, for example, found that 48 percent of patients wanted help with home safety from their physician, 45 percent wanted help with financial concerns, and 30 percent were looking for help with mental or emotional problems.[21] Chances are these figures represent far higher expectations than physicians are aware of or prepared to deal with. Yet, if you learn what consumers' problems and concerns are, you can select the problems to address, at least, and the solutions to offer in influencing their expectations: you will have a chance to make good decisions. Ignorance of their expectations on the other hand, may leave you unable to help and your loyalist prospects disgruntled.

It may be equally important to learn what consumers are *not* looking for. Such knowledge can keep you from investing in the delivery of benefits they don't want. It is particularly helpful if you have heard about some popular program or if some expert has advised you to implement some program—but no consumers have suggested it. At a minimum, ask your target consumers if they want the benefit you have in mind, at the price you would need to set, and if they would *prefer* getting it from you versus merely liking the idea in general.

In seeking to learn what consumers are looking for, find out how they define loyalty. *What would it mean to them for your organization to be loyal to its customers?* As later discussion of the Loyalty Marketing Wheel will show, it is essential that consumers perceive your loyalty to them if you expect to achieve, maintain, and mine their loyalty to you. Discovering the expectations of desired individual consumers and populations will both pinpoint the persons you may be able to convert to loyalty and provide a basis for estimating the cost of their loyalty to you.

What are their specific expectations (if they are loyal consumers) with repeated encounters? Do they expect to be able to reach the same familiar (and well-liked) member service representative, for example, or to see the same physician each time they make a visit? Do they have a high interest in receiving information from you?[7] How do they rate you as a source of the information they want? How does your plan rate compared to other plans; how do you compare with other hospitals, physicians, and nurses?[22]

Although drawing such insights from current and prospective customers is essential in the pursuit of informed loyalty, it is not enough. Consumers are notoriously limited in identifying their own concerns, particularly those needs and wishes that may be subconscious, semiconscious, or embarrassing to mention. Normally, they are incapable of identifying benefits that they know of no way to gain, for example, or of articulating unfamiliar ideas on ways for benefits to be delivered. You should supplement the insights you gain from consumers with ideas from your own imagination and your understanding of what is possible. Then subsequently, you need to validate those ideas through concept and pilot testing with consumers.

Even before you serve particular consumers, it may help if you obtain health risk and problem information from them. Conducting a health risk assessment before the plan member or patient makes a first visit can suggest the consumers who are most at risk, with the greatest potential to gain from a healthcare relationship with you.[23] Armed with this information, you can create for these consumers—or with them—a long-term plan for dealing with the health risks identified, thus preparing the way for a long-term, mutually beneficial relationship.

Just as it is essential to learn consumers' expectations for each encounter with you—the *difference* the consumers expect and hope you will make through particular customer contacts—so it is essential to learn their expectations of a loyal relationship: the differences they expect and prefer it to make in their lives. Why do they expect and prefer to see the same physician each time they need care, for example, or prefer to see the first one available? Why do they expect and prefer to be able to talk to the same member service representative or personal nurse counselor every time they have a question about the health plan?

Consumer expectations regarding loyal relationships are not simply givens, however, for you to identify. One of the challenges in marketing is to *influence* consumer expectations through planning the value to promise, deliver, and report to them. Expectations need to be *managed* as part of managing the relationship itself, because everything you do for consumers and say to them can affect their expectations and influence their perceptions of value received. The learning step merely begins the task of managing expectations[24] (more in chapter 3).

4. Information that Helps Build Loyalty

The previously listed information is useful primarily in selecting the consumers to pursue and in deciding on loyalty strategies; other kinds of information, however, are likely to be useful in day-to-day efforts to achieve and maintain consumer loyalty. First of all is information about consumers (and household/family members) *as persons*. The more familiar you are with them as individuals (and the more familiar they are with you), the better chance you have of accomplishing your loyalty goals.[25] Specific information is useful in each of the loyalty marketing steps that follow.

The development of databases on consumer populations, and dossiers on individuals, has been widely accepted in marketing in general and in the health sector in particular. The maintenance of patient and enrollee records is required by law; consumers expect it, and it is of great practical value. The key to developing loyalty databases lies in including personal information about interests, values, concerns, and expectations that can enable you to deliver added value. Limited records of clinical and service outcomes and insurance coverage offer little useful loyalty information.

What critical incidents in the past have been of great benefit or heavy cost to consumers? What specific value effects have particular experiences had, and how did consumers feel about them? Have specific individuals had good or bad experiences, and good efforts at recovery—or bad ones brought about by service failures?[26] What special treatment would they like on a regular basis, or what special favors would they wish you to do for them at particular contacts?[27] Patterns of answers to such questions enable you to improve your value delivery in general; idiosyncratic answers from individuals allow you to customize your value delivery for the greatest positive effect on loyalty.

What specific benefits and costs do prospective and current customers perceive as arising from certain service structures and processes?[28] What natural and predictable needs and concerns can you expect over time from their lifecycle transitions, and where are particular identified consumers located in their lifecycles? If you can use such information to *anticipate and proact* to needs, problems, and wishes, that is, if you can *surprise* them with unexpected value, you will be well ahead of your purely reactive rivals.[29]

You should aim for an *intimacy* of relevant knowledge and understanding of the consumers whom you wish to be loyal.[30] From current customers, you should learn the ways they have found to maximize the benefits they've gained from you, in encounters and from your relationship, their means of coping with medical demands, physical problems, and administrative hassles—the ways they have found to minimize inconveniences and costs. You can pass along what you have learned to new converts, enabling them to gain as much value now as your veteran loyalists have gained earlier.

Because you will be communicating with consumers about the value you promise, reminding them of the value they have gained, promoting their return of value, and recognizing them for the value they have returned, you should learn their preferred approaches to communicating. What are their preferences for timing, the "proper place," and the "best way" to be contacted? What matters do they want to be told about? What sources of information (individuals and organizations) do they find most helpful and credible, and for what reasons? Although you can identify the media and sources that actually work best as you move ahead in your loyalty marketing, having some up-front ideas should help.

Because you anticipate delivering, communicating, tracking, and reminding consumers of your value later on in the loyalty marketing process, it helps if you can learn not only the benefits they are after, but the *measures* of benefit most meaningful to them. Identifying the kinds of benefits they will agree to track for themselves will help you in developing your tracking system. Tracing patterns of consumer preference can guide your overall tracking and reminder systems, and noting individual preferences can enable you to customize to such preferences where possible and to optimize their subsequent effect.

And because you are preparing to manage, communicate, track, and remind consumers of the value you anticipate delivering, it is essential that you identify specific value effects that consumers want and that you can deliver *at the outset.* Then stick with them. Strive to avoid the strong tendency to back away from enduring quality of life value as soon as possible and deal instead with the structures, processes, and even clinical outcomes that we think of as somewhat controllable, in contrast to *value*—that idiosyncratic and uncontrollable difference to their lives that consumers perceive.

In his classic work on healthcare quality, for example, Donabedian noted that after structure, process, and outcome comes "valuation." He realized that patient valuations vary widely regarding the things that providers do for and to them, and the importance that valuation holds in the overall quality of care delivered. Because it is not possible to predict or manage the value that consumers place on the "during" and "enduring" effects of care, Donabedian did not include consumer valuation in his approach to defining and assessing quality.[28]

The pursuit of consumer loyalty, in contrast to the assessment or management of quality, places value as the key dimension. If the right value is not identified in the first place—the specific value effects that consumers are after in particular encounters and in loyal relationships—success in achieving, maintaining, and mining loyalty will come purely by chance. In one dramatic example, when consumers were asked to put a dollar value on a prenatal ultrasound test, they came up with a figure ten times as much as the charge that prevailed. Knowing they had a healthy baby was worth that much more than worrying.[31]

To illustrate in a simple transaction mode, consider a physician group that is focusing on increasing the loyalty of its patients, but only as customers. The group conducts some market research and finds through factor analysis that the key to significant improvement in patient satisfaction and loyalty is "access." Analysis reveals that this one factor accounts for 67 percent of all variation in satisfaction and loyalty among current patients, and for 50 percent of the variation in preferences among prospective patients.

The group practice's marketing experts (and associate and assistant experts) home in on "access" as the principal focus for loyalty enhancement. They decide that the best way to enhance consumer access is to offer evening and weekend hours, and to add locations closer to the consumers' homes. They arrange delivery of this improvement in their offer to consumers, at an additional cost of $650,000 a year. They promise, deliver, track, and remind patients and prospects of the improved "access" they are delivering.

But they are making at least two serious mistakes. First, "access" is neither a value, an outcome, a process, or even a structure: it is a formless general category—a "factor"—that summarizes a number of possible specifics. One of the problems with factor analysis is its translation of practical specifics into "academic" generalities. But the key to "rolling the value wheel" at this stage is *specifics*—hard, manageable, concrete improvements and distinctions in value.

Perhaps the patients of this group practice simply want shorter waits for appointments, for example: that is what *they* mean by improved access. Or perhaps they want locations closer to their workplace, on public transportation lines, or with parking readily available and free. Maybe they mean lower deductibles and copayments for particular services. They might even mean that they would like the practice to replace the person who answers the phone with a snarl and puts them on hold.

Without a handle on the particulars, identifying access as a major problem or opportunity area means nothing—and is dangerous. The practice's investment in expanding its hours could be a waste of time and money. Translating into specifics is essential; ways to do so when consumers themselves cite vague factors, such as access, will be discussed in the next section, on "Ways to Learn What Consumers Want."

The lack of specifics also means that consumer definitions may be spread across different accessibility need segments. Some people define access in terms of office locations, others in terms of appointments, others in hours (finding parking, for example, or having to feed the meter). Unless marketers find out what each consumer means by access, these needs segments will not be identified. And unless these segments are identified, marketers will not know how many consumers will be won over by an offer of added locations, and how many need some other offer improvement. They will not be able to decide whether to go for one or more segments, nor will they know how.

This lack of specificity, with its problems, applies to all of the generalized dimensions that consumers may cite or researchers use to summarize "factors." Such vague summarizations of data risk turning distinct consumer segments into a homogenized and useless average. A set of consumers may reflect a bimodal distribution in terms of their wants, so that by averaging the distribution, marketers come up with an offer neither mode will accept. One mode might want a $25 per visit price, for example, and anything much more than that will turn them away. The other may think that any visit price lower than $50 indicates an incompetent provider. The marketer who averages these distinct preferences to offer a $37.50 visit will likely attract no patients.

The second mistake is to overlook the specific *value* that causes a particular vague dimension, specific structure, or process to be desired by consumers. Suppose that a prompter appointment schedule was the specific process improvement that consumers wanted in the earlier case. If the marketers were to go no further than this, they could well cause the group practice to invest in new software and appointment systems and staff, costing perhaps hundreds of thousands of dollars to deliver that explicit process improvement.

But what if the reason consumers wanted prompter appointments was anxiety when their children were sick and could not wait a week or more to see the doctor? What if their anxiety could have been alleviated, in 90 percent of the cases, by providing a nurse counselor to talk to them by phone and a self-care manual costing $10 a copy? In that case, the ultimate value they were after might have been delivered at a fraction of the cost and it would have done a better job (by phone for that 90 percent and by a walk-in arrangement for the other 10 percent). Without a precise identification of the value that drove those consumer requests for improvement, only the option of a new appointment system would have even been considered.

Once the ultimate *value* has been identified, it can be used as the first focus of management's design efforts to figure out its specific delivery. Your best option can be chosen based on its effectiveness, promptness, and efficiency in delivering the precise value desired. As soon as the value delivery method has been selected, it can be consciously managed in ways that promote the delivery of that value. Nurse triage counselors can be trained for expertise in alleviating the anxiety of callers. Their performance appraisals, salaries, and bonuses can be made to reflect their success in delivering the prime value.

Precise, meaningful value can then be promised to prospective patients or plan members, both to clarify the benefits you will deliver to them and to add to their appreciation of them. Value can then be tracked to ensure that it is perceived as well as delivered, and reminders of specific value benefits can be used to heighten consumers' awareness, appreciation, and attribution of their advantages gained in maintaining a loyal relationship with you.

5. Loyalty Status Up Front

For your accurate assessment of the situation and its challenge, it helps if you identify the current status of loyalty among the consumers you are targeting for attention. Both the extent of their loyalty, if any, and its current object are likely to be valuable to know. You can place consumers on specific rungs of a "ladder" of loyalty, for example, starting at the bottom with those who are "inert" in the market, not interacting with anyone, and "shoppers," those who are interacting but with no one in particular in their frequent, sometimes whimsical, changes in providers. Next would be the "splitters": those who take their business to a small number of organizations, including yours. The next rung would be the "leaners": consumers who split, but come to you more often than to others. You could call the next group "clients": those who almost always come to you but who limit themselves solely to customer interactions. At the top are your "champions," those who are wholly committed to you and who contribute in roles that go beyond mere customer activities.

You could characterize entire populations on a loyalty ladder, but you would have to include more lower rungs: shoppers and splitters who do not include you among the organizations they do business with, as well as leaners toward your rivals, plus *their* clients and champions. In general, you would use such a ladder to target consumers only after you exhausted the potential of everyone doing at least some business with you. "Converting" consumers who are loyal to your rivals normally is much more difficult to do than converting the shoppers and leaners who already interact with you.

For health plans, loyalty ladders are much shorter. They include no shoppers, splitters, or leaners, because people are either members of your plan or not. They certainly include your rivals' clients and champions, as well as some "inerts" who have not yet joined any plan, plus your own clients and champions. Plans may well characterize loyalty in terms of a membership time line as well as on the strength of customers' preferences and reenrollment intentions.

In addition to helping you choose your consumers of special interest, and indicating the situation among those consumers, the levels at which you place consumers on the loyalty ladder will provide the basis for monitoring and evaluating your success in moving them up toward your champions' level. Although tracking the numbers of consumers as well as the types and the value of their contributions will tell you more than their placement on the ladder ever can, the ladder provides a good way to summarize the amount of change you have made in consumer loyalty (more on this in chapter 6).

Ways to Learn What Consumers Want

A book like this has no room in it to describe all of your options in gathering the kinds of information already discussed. No single book could cover the full range of possibilities. What I can do is to suggest some particularly useful approaches and to cite references for you to pursue for more detailed discussions of them. I also indicate why I think each approach to gaining information can be particularly useful in loyalty-learning marketing research (in contrast to transaction-focused applications) and the means to make each approach useful.

Non-Arms-Length Approaches

First I recommend that you consider learning techniques other than those of traditional survey research. If you already have any sort of relationship with the consumers you target for loyalty, getting them more intimately involved in your learning efforts will, by itself, help promote loyalty in addition to enabling you to gain information. Seating them on the same side of the table (literally, if possible, but at least figuratively) and working on "solving the problem" of ways to deliver more value to themselves and help you gain their loyalty will promote early on a sense of partnership.

When you are dealing with a small number of loyalty prospects, you may be able to include all of them in a joint planning, problem-solving, decision-making process. When the numbers are too large, you can include a representative sample for the inferential base you need to extrapolate your research data. This effort should also give you a small set of precommitted converts who will likely use the offer they helped design. Then they can promote the conversion of their peers by "spreading the word."

The challenge of designing an irresistible loyalty offer may be approached with your group as a common problem that calls for joint planning and brainstorming. A slightly less intimate approach is "virtual negotiation," in which both parties sit down at the table but on different sides.[32] You ask them what it will take to make them loyal and use what they tell you to design the loyalty offer, coupled with your own ideas that they can validate for you during "negotiation" sessions.

Another group process amenable to identifying priority values among consumers is the Nominal Group technique.[33] Although it is used mainly in internal planning, this technique can be adapted to your loyalty learning effort. It consists of first asking each individual member of a group (usually of eight or so) or groups (as many as you can accommodate) to write up a list of the most important benefits and costs they see as potentially or currently involved in a relationship with a plan or provider. You might ask them to spend ten minutes on a list of physical health benefits, for example, then another ten on the psychological/social/emotional benefits. You will usually have to explain what you mean by a benefit and a cost, so that they don't simply discuss general factors or structure and process isues like those described earlier.

Once each person has compiled a list (and the list is made before any discussion is allowed, except with the group facilitator), each person in each group is invited, in turn, to name one item on his or her list as a "recorder" in each group puts the items on a display board. When everyone's list is exhausted, facilitators guide discussions to clarify and prioritize the display board list, putting the group to a vote if discussion fails to produce a consensus list of top value items.

A recent variation on this technique starts with individual dyads of consumers, each creating a list that the two discuss until they reach consensus on the most important three to five items. Each dyad then meets with another dyad until the four reach consensus. This is repeated with four times four, eight times eight, and larger groups if necessary, until the entire group has reached consensus.[34] Both this and the Nominal Group Process are useful primarily when consensus of a homogeneous group, such as employees in a single firm or union, or members of an organization, are involved and a single loyalty offer is to be made to the entire group.

When your task is to estimate the value or the probability of something, or to provide an estimate or forecast of any parameter, the Delphi technique is often recommended. Basically, this requires assembling or obtaining agreement from a set of well-informed stakeholder participants, internal or external as appropriate. All are asked for their individual estimates or forecasts, which are averaged and reported back to them. Those whose figures are comparative outliers are asked to explain their figures or revise them. Participants are then asked to reconsider their figures compared to the average and in light of the explanations of the outliers. Eventually, all participants usually reach a consensus; if that is impossible, an average "vote" is used.[35]

Individual in-depth interviews and focus groups can also be used as less than arms-length means of learning about consumer loyalty. The point is to make the methods use dialogues and conversations rather than unilateral collections of data. Giving consumers a sense that they are aiding a joint effort to improve the value you deliver to them and to promote their satisfaction and loyalty can give the loyalty marketing initiative a running start, whereas simply collecting information may be annoying or perceived as an invasion of privacy.[36]

In effect, these exercises are asking consumers to teach you the best ways to serve them. As Peppers and Rogers point out, this can give you three personal contacts with each consumer to promote loyalty as well as learn about it: (1) asking them to delineate specific benefits or costs that concern them; (2) telling them what you have learned and asking them for validation; and then (3) telling them what you plan to do about their concerns, perhaps eliciting their feedback to be sure your plans are on the right track.[37]

Laddering

Laddering is a technique specifically suited to learning about the values that consumers are after from encounters and relationships. Originally part of the "reportorial grid" method,[38] laddering[39] works, first, by asking consumers three questions: "What makes a good health plan or provider?" "How do you choose one over others?" and "What makes you want to be loyal to one or another?" Because consumers are just as loathe to discuss their personal values as most managers are to work with them, the answers they give are likely to consist of structures, processes, or "attributes" (i.e., their subjective opinions and value judgments about particular plans and providers attributed as if they were the objective characteristics of those plans and providers and not simply their own opinions).

When consumers describe their wants or ways of choosing in terms of structure and process *factors*, laddering asks them to move "up the ladder of abstraction" to their reasons for finding such factors compelling. Interviewers can ask, "What does that do for you?" or "Why is that important to you?" to get consumers to think more in terms of specific benefits and costs than of structures and processes. When consumers reach clear benefits, such as how they are made to feel and effects on their quality of life, the questioning about the particular factor can stop. When all factors have been identified and "laddered up" to their underlying values, a values map is constructed showing the number of factors that lead to a specific number of values.

The map will first show the number of values engaged in a particular encounter or relationship decision. It will then show the number of factors linked to each of the values identified—with the assumption that the number of factors linked to each value roughly signals those values more important to the particular choice examined to the particular interviewee consumer(s). (The laddering process is designed for individual in-person interviews, but I have obtained useful results in group discussions, via fax and Internet, as well.)

Because personal values, in terms of the benefits consumers desire from particular products and services, are often subconscious or even unconscious, hypnosis is a technique used with some success in bringing them out. Focus groups in which all participants have volunteered to be hypnotized before the discussions have been used to identify the reasons behind brand preferences when the benefits have not been obvious. Emotional memories and dimensions of experience revealed under hypnosis have helped in designing marketing campaigns.[40]

Although it is not officially part of the laddering technique, I have long used a reverse approach: descending the ladder rather than climbing up. In some cases, consumers have identified factors other than structure and process items as key to a loyal relationship. These are usually subjective attributes, and I've asked them how they can tell if a (plan or provider) is (competent, friendly, efficient, caring, trustworthy)—whatever they have identified as the key attributes. Your organization or plan cannot deliver such attributes by simply telling your staff to be more competent or friendly, and so on: these are subjective consumer judgments, and only by getting consumers themselves to tell you what they mean can you learn how to deliver those values by changing specific structures and processes.

Once the technique has identified the key values, the interviewer can sound out participating consumers to validate the findings. This is done first by reporting the value map to participants (perhaps showing it to them) and asking them if the values that appear to be most important indeed are so to them. Later on, when the new or improved loyalty offer has been designed, the design is pretested with consumers by asking them if the design is what they had in mind, and would it, indeed, represent an irresistible offer.

Survey Techniques

When close group approaches or individual interviews are not feasible, a number of different survey approaches can work well. A sentence completion approach, for example, asks consumers to complete sentences such as this one: "If I had a good relationship with (hospital, plan, physician, etc.), I would enjoy (being, having, feeling) more/less. . . ." (The same can be used for encounters, with the word "visit," "stay," or "encounter" used instead of "relationship.") A variation on this approach asks about good relationships (or encounters) that consumers have had, and puts the question in the past tense: "When I had . . . ," and so forth.

Importance/Performance Analysis

A long-used and widely successful technique in market research, normally used for transaction marketing but easily adaptable to loyalty, is called Importance/Performance Analysis.[41,42] Initial discussions aim at identifying the key value dimensions that consumers look for *in a relationship* with a plan or provider. (Any of the above techniques can be used for this.) Then the persons interviewed or surveyed rate each value on its importance to them. One approach is to ask them to distribute 100 points among the values.[43]

Once participants have identified and ranked or rated the importance of key benefit or value dimensions, they are asked to rank and to rate a set of competing plans or providers, including your organization, on each of these dimensions, and finally to rate and rank their overall preference. Both rating and ranking provide insights. Rating suggests the relative advantages that consumers see for options on an absolute scale, indicating possible room for your improvement; both the importance rating and the gap between your option and the best-rated option tell you the importance of working on one value in contrast to the others. Ranking gives you a sense of where you stand: you want to be ranked first regardless of your absolute score.

In general, few survey techniques can tell you all you want to know about loyalty and value dimensions. Close-ended questions, in particular, are poorly suited to this purpose. You will want to use open-ended questions and probe consumers until they divulge the kind of information you would get from the laddering technique: not only what the key values are, but consumers' thoughts on the structure, process, and outcome factors most likely to deliver those values. You will not want to rely on what they tell you, but you certainly want to start there. Statistical correlation can often yield insights into the dimensions of true importance when consumer-reported input is incomplete.[44]

When gauging consumers' loyalty, it is possible to ask them to indicate their personal position on the loyalty ladder. You can ask questions about their knowledge and awareness of your organization, with total ignorance putting them at the bottom and some awareness just above that. Asking them to indicate their attitudes toward you, at levels of "interest," "willingness to try," and "intention to try next time," would show higher levels of potential for loyalty although no loyalty as such. Identifying those who "have tried," are "satisfied," "prefer" you, and voice a "commitment" to you would complete a loyalty ladder based on self-reporting.

Unlike consumer satisfaction, which has been subject to literally hundreds of survey techniques and scales, loyalty has barely had the surface scratched as a subject for survey. Intentions to return and recommend are commonly used but often without the inclusion of an indication of preference or strength of preference. Asking if a patient would return to your practice or hospital, without asking whether the consumer would choose it over all other options, results in a poor gauge of loyalty.

In any case, the best gauge of loyalty is not an expression of attitudes or intentions, but the consumer's actual behavior. Consumer behavior that contributes to your performance is, first, the best indicator of loyalty. Although inertia may cause retention, behavior has the added advantage of contributing value and more meaningful loyalty. Finally, contributory behavior seems to strengthen as well as to indicate the loyalty you're looking for[17] (more in chapter 7).

Observation Techniques

In addition to the individual and group approaches with consumers telling you directly what they value, some indirect techniques are available to supplement what consumers can and will say. With many values residing at subconscious or unconscious levels, it is helpful to have a secondary source of insight based on observations of consumer behavior. A "mystery shopper" masquerading as a patient or plan member, for example, can carefully scrutinize, record, and report on the consumer experiences you are actually delivering. Mystery shoppers cannot be relied on to report value delivered, or to discuss relationships, but they can be helpful with encounters. Consumers themselves have been trained to be mystery shoppers, adding to their value as customers.[45]

A technique called "empathic" observation can also be used to gauge consumer experiences with encounters. Trained observers watch consumers as they are served, looking for body language and other indicators of problems, concerns, or issues that consumers may be unaware of or hesitant to mention. The technique found that surgeons relying on a TV monitor to view their progress during laparascopic surgery were unaware of the frequency (though brief in each instance) with which the circulating nurses interrupted them, breaking their line of vision. The surgeons never mentioned the problem, although a headset monitor fixed in front of their eyes subsequently made them a lot happier.[46]

Using another example, observations of consumers for injury prevention and stress reduction, at home or at work, can supplement survey and other self-reporting approaches. Home health providers, peers, and occupational health providers can document observations that reveal facts and inferences that consumers never report or even notice directly. Knowledge from such observations may greatly enhance the scope of benefits that you can offer or can serve as the basis for pleasant surprises that promote high satisfaction and loyalty.

Humana uses a system that records and categorizes all information, complaints, praise, or other comments from callers as a means of finding out those benefits and costs that seem to have the most value effect on consumers.[47] A similar approach records the information that Web site visitors are downloading as an indication of the concerns important to them, in case they are identifying value problems they have not reported. It is wise to offer multiple means by which you can talk with consumers and they can talk to you, from suggestion boxes to hot lines to "town meetings," in addition to multiple research techniques, in order to get the full picture of values important to consumers.[48]

Looking Forward

The purpose of learning about loyalty is to provide you with the marketing intelligence essential for carrying out the next steps in loyalty marketing. The knowledge you've acquired should contribute to each of the subsequent steps. Your stock of knowledge provides the foundation for management of the design, development, and delivery of value; for expertise in promising value offered; and for success in tracking it and reminding loyalty prospects about it. Thinking forward to ways in which you will use your learning capability and the knowledge it leads to can help improve your planning and your continued implementation of the learning process.

For example, as you conduct focus group discussions and other techniques involving groups of prospects, consider asking your own staff and decision makers to observe the process—at least on videotape. By involving the employees who will ultimately be delivering value in pursuit of loyalty and the decision makers who will ultimately decide whether to approve and finance the effort, you will greatly promote their acceptance—even enthusiasm—in carrying out their roles. Your challenge in devising any value delivery proposal is to make so irresistible the value you promise and deliver, track, and remind, that the consumers will eagerly accept your offer and become your loyal clients and champions. Equally important is the challenge of making your proposed initiative irresistible to the internal decision makers, who must approve and commit the resources needed to carry it out, and to the staff, whose enthusiasm in delivering your offer will make an enormous difference in the success of your initiative. The more you keep both purposes in mind, the better.

To illustrate, I've heard of one organization that was having trouble getting the CEO to release funds for service improvements. Concerned managers arranged for a group of customers to visit the facility and meet with the CEO, and during the meeting those customers voiced their concerns and complaints regarding service. The CEO immediately released the funds. Nothing like going right to the source for solving the problem!

There are limits, of course, to what you can find out through any market research techniques. Assuming causality from correlation is a common problem in healthcare, especially when the timing of the events is not clear. Do attitudes *cause* behavior, for example, or is it the other way around?[49] Information that consumers report may be affected by any number of conscious and unconscious factors. Evaluation after the fact should always be used to validate any up-front learning (more about this in chapter 6).

Figure 1-2   Learning Connections

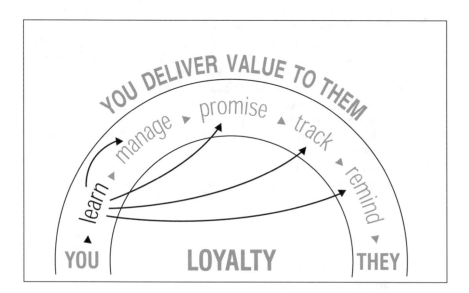

Action Recommendations

✓ Identify the types and value of benefits you can hope to gain from loyal relationships with selected sets of consumers, specifying what they would do to deliver such benefits to you. (**Suggested:** the Nominal Group technique and joint planning approach) _____

✓ Estimate the probability of achieving such benefits from each set of consumers considered as possible targets for loyalty investment. (**Suggested:** Delphi technique involving internal stakeholders—possibly consumers as well—and joint planning) _____

✓ Select the sets of consumer prospects to focus on based on your estimate of value times your estimate of the probability of achieving that value. (**Suggested:** Delphi or joint planning) _____

✓ Determine the quality of life benefits your selected consumers expect and hope for from a relationship with your kind of organization and the importance of such benefits to them. (**Suggested:** focus groups, surveys, and joint planning) _____

✓ Determine consumers' perceptions of your organization compared to their perceptions of rival organizations in terms of the ability to deliver such benefits, based on past performance and perceived intentions. (**Suggested:** importance/performance analysis and joint planning) _____

✓ Select the consumers who show the greatest potential for loyalty, list your current advantages and disadvantages relative to rival organizations, and the benefits and costs to work on in improving your loyalty value proposition. (**Suggested:** Nominal Group technique and joint planning) _____

✓ Devise your unique loyalty value proposition describing your intended performance value gained from selected consumers' loyalty, and the quality of life value you will deliver to them in order to gain that loyalty value. (**Suggested:** Nominal Group technique and joint planning) _____

✓ Create databases on consumer segments and dossiers on individuals, as appropriate, based on the value to be gained from each segment and individual and the value of such information in realizing that value. (**Suggested:** Delphi for estimating value) _____

✓ Use these loyalty learning techniques to promote your relations with selected consumers as well as to learn about such individuals wherever possible. _____

References

1. MacStravic, S. 1998. "Who's Your Best Customer?" *Managed Care Quarterly* 6, no. 3 (summer): 1–6.
2. Huppertz, J. 1998. "Turning Consumer Data Into Marketing Strategy." *Alliance for Healthcare Strategy and Marketing Annual Conference Proceedings* (1 April): 397–416.
3. Duboff, R., and L. Sherer. 1997. "Customized Customer Loyalty." *Marketing Management* 6, no. 2 (summer): 20–27.
4. Rosenberg, L., and J. Czepiel. 1984. "A Marketing Approach to Customer Retention." *Journal of Consumer Marketing* 1 (2): 11–24.
5. Christopher, M., A. Payne, and D. Ballantyne. 1991. *Relationship Marketing: Bringing Quality, Customer Service, and Marketing Together.* Oxford: Butterworth-Heinemann.
6. Woodside, A., L. Frey, and R. T. Daly. 1989. "Linking Service Quality, Customer Satisfaction and Behavioral Intention." *Journal of Health Care Marketing* 9, no. 4 (December): 5–17.
7. Whiteley, R., and D. Hessan. 1996. *Customer Centered Growth: Five Strategies for Building Competitive Advantage,* pp. 1–13. Reading, MA: Addison-Wesley.

8. Baron, G. 1996. "The Four Stages of a Loyal Business Relationship." *Marketing News* 30, no. 19 (9 September): 7.

9. "Analysis Looks at Member Loyalty for Health Benefit Plans." *Healthcare Strategy Alert* (January 1998): 8.

10. "What Makes a Person Loyal to a Hospital?" *Strategies* (newsletter) First Marketing Company, West Linn, OR. 3, no. 3 (undated): 2–3.

11. Ferguson, T. 1996. *Health Online: How to Find Information, Support Groups, and Self-Help Communities in Cyberspace.* Reading, MA: Addison-Wesley.

12. Kertesz, L. 1998. "Standing By Their Plan." *Modern Healthcare* (20 April): 108–12.

13. Jensen, J. 1989. "Patients Who Choose Their Hospital Are More Satisfied." *Modern Healthcare* (28 July): 66–68.

14. Scotti, D., and P. G. Bonner. 1985. "On the Use of Attitudinal Data to Predict Reenrollment Behavior: How Good Are Subscribers' Intentions?" In *1985 Group Health Proceedings,* pp. 393–402. Washington, DC: Group Health Association of America.

15. Griffin, J. 1995. *Customer Loyalty.* New York: Lexington Books.

16. Lackman, R., and S. Noy. 1996. "Reaction of Salaried Physicians to Hospital Decline." *Health Services Research* 31, no. 2 (June): 171–90.

17. Fisk, T., C. Brown, K. Cannizzaro, and B. Naftal. 1990. "Creating Patient Satisfaction and Loyalty." *Journal of Health Care Marketing* 10, no. 2 (June): 5–15.

18. Bell, C. 1994. *Customers as Partners: Building Relationships That Last.* San Francisco: Berrett-Koehler.

19. Hornberger, J., and L. Lenert. 1996. "Variations Among Quality-of-Life Surveys." *Medical Care* 34, no. 12 (December, Supplement): S23-S33.

20. "Can't Get No Customer Satisfaction?" *Quality Digest* 16, no. 8 (August 1996): 13.

21. Lynch, W. 1996. "Demand Management in Healthcare." Strategic Research Conference, Chicago, 30 May.

22. "Consumers Seek Advice from Registered Nurses When Making Health Care Choices." *Health Care Strategic Managment* 16, no. 5 (May 1998): 6.

23. Jahnke, R., and N. Faass. 1998. "Health Assessment Is the Gateway to Improved Outcomes Across All Populations." *Inside Preventive Care* 4 (April): 1, 9–11.

24. Baker, S. 1998. *Managing Patient Expectations,* p. 37. San Francisco: Jossey-Bass.

25. Derlega, V., et al. 1987. "Self-Disclosure and Relationship Development." In *Interpersonal Process: New Directions in Communications Research,* edited by M. Roloff and G. Miller. London: Sage.

26. Bitner, M. J., B. Booms, and M. S. Tetreault. 1989. "Critical Incidents in Service Encounters." In *Designing a Winning Service Strategy,* edited by M. J. Bitner and L. Crosby, pp. 98–99. Chicago: American Marketing Association.

27. Bonoma, T. 1994. "Marketing's Colors: Al's Gas Town." *Marketing Management* 3 (2): 17–24.

28. Donabedian, A. 1980. *The Definition of Quality and Approaches to its Assessment,* pp. 3-31. Chicago: Health Administration Press.

29. Morath, J. 1998. "Beyond Utilization Control: Managing Care With Customers." *Managed Care Quarterly* 6, no. 3 (summer): 46–52.

30. Bell, C., and R. Zemke. 1992. *Managing Knock Your Socks Off Service.* New York: AMACOM.

31. Berwick, D., and M. Weinstein. 1985. "What Do Patients Value?" *Medical Care* 23, no. 7 (July): 881.

32. MacStravic, S. 1998. "Virtual Negotiation in Health Care Marketing." *Strategic Health Care Marketing* 16, no. 5 (May): 3–5.

33. Delbecq, A., A. Van de Ven, and D. Gustafson. 1975. *Group Techniques for Program Planning,* pp. 1–39, 83–107. Glenview, IL: Scott, Foresman.

34. Blanchard, K., and M. O'Connor. 1997. *Managing by Values.* San Francisco: Berrett-Koehler.

35. Raider, A. 1998. "Closed Loop Marketing." *The Cowles Report on Database Marketing* 7, no. 8 (August): 1, 10.

36. "Repersonalizing Health Care by Mass Customizing It on a One-to-One Basis." *Health Care Strategic Management* 15, no. 7 (July 1997): 13.

37. Peppers, D., and M. Rogers. 1994. "Welcome to the 1:1 Future." *Marketing Tools* 1, no. 1 (April/May): 4–7.

38. Reynolds, R., and L. Jameson. 1984. "Image Representations." In *Perceived Quality: How Customers View Stores and Merchandise,* edited by J. Jacoby and J. Olson, pp. 115-38. New York: Lexington Books.

39. Myers, J. 1996. "Positioning Based On Laddering." In *Segmentation and Positioning for Strategic Marketing Decisions,* pp. 263–82. Chicago: American Marketing Association.

40. Fellman, M. W. 1998. "Mesmerizing Method Gets Real Results." *Marketing News* 32, no. 15 (20 July): 1, 38.

41. Martilla, J., and J. James. 1977. "Importance-Performance Analysis." *Journal of Health Care Marketing* 5 (1): 77–79.

42. Hawes, J., and C. Rao. 1985. "Using Importance-Performance Analysis to Develop Health Care Marketing Strategies." *Journal of Health Care Marketing* 5 (4): 19–25.

43. Yavas, U., and D. Shemwell. 1996. "Competing for Patients and Profit." *Journal of Health Care Marketing* 16, no. 2 (summer): 30–37.

44. Neslin, S. 1983. "Designing New Outpatient Features." *Journal of Health Care Marketing* 3, no. 3 (summer): 8–21.

45. "Health Care Mata Hari." *Hospitals & Health Networks* (20 April 1997): 46–48.

46. Leonard, D., and J. Rayport. 1997. "Spark Innovation Through Empathic Design." *Harvard Business Review* 75, no. 6 (November/December): 102–13.

47. Bulgar, D., and S. Sloate. 1997. "Return on Investment–Based One-on-One Program." In *Future Vision: Technology and Healthcare Marketing.* Chicago: Alliance for Healthcare Strategy and Marketing Conference Proceedings.

48. Baum, N. 1992. *Marketing Your Clinical Practice.* Gaithersburg, MD: Aspen.

49. Skinner, B. F. 1972. *Beyond Freedom and Dignity.* New York: Free Press.

MANAGING VALUE DELIVERY

Figure 2-1

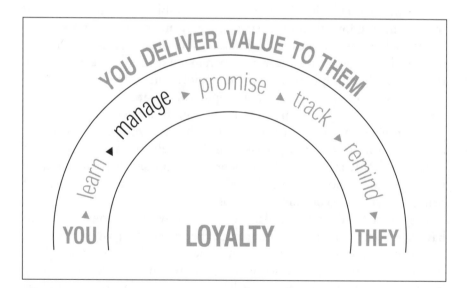

O NCE YOU have completed the learning discussed in the preceding
chapter, you are ready to translate your knowledge into the value
you will deliver. This value may lie in a brand new offer, a new
plan or option, a new service or program, or a significant improvement
in a current offer. You have four tasks: (1) select the consumers who will

receive your value offer, (2) design the offer, (3) develop the system to deliver it, and (4) deliver it when consumers come for it. Although you decide on loyalty prospects and you design and develop the offer before the consumers come—and then you deliver it after they arrive—all four tasks are presented here. They are too closely related not to keep them together, even though the "promise" step (chapter 3) takes place before the actual delivery.

Deciding on Loyalty Prospects

Loyalty marketing is more expensive than transaction marketing, so it should be used selectively and prudently. Not all consumers are logical prospects. You may not want some to be loyal, and some may not want to be loyal. It may take too much trouble and expense to go after some compared to their potential value to you. On the other hand, you may have to start by attracting as many consumers as you can and then selecting which to "keep" after you have had some experience with them (more in chapter 6).

It is wise to select loyalty prospects by combining the potential gain from achieving loyalty among particular consumers and the probability of such achievement. The learning process should have given you enough information to estimate these two parameters, so that selection will require simply multiplying the two and prioritizing options.

The best prospects normally are people who are at least potentially interested in a loyal relationship and who see significant benefit possibilities for themselves in such a relationship. Consumers who prefer to "shop" and enjoy variety for its own sake can be deselected and reserved for transaction-only attention.[1] Consumers who appear reluctant or unable to reciprocate, who are unmotivated to return value to you as part of being loyal, can also be eliminated from the prospect list.[2]

In general, loyalty is pursued more successfully among consumers who have had some contact with your organization in the past, so that you have some records on them and can place them at the "shopper" level of loyalty or above. (Many who have great potential value to you may be at the more or less "inert" levels, and they will invariably be more difficult to approach. For them, a better option is to aim for some initial transaction before you invest in the full loyalty marketing process.)

Especially promising are consumers who have had some contact with you (the more recent the better) *and* are at the top of the satisfaction rating scale when they rate you. Those at the top of the scale are likely to be at least twice as willing as inert consumers to become loyal. Working to bring up one level those already next to the top will yield more value than aiming to convert those who are lower down.[3]

Your selection effort should conclude with the most promising numbers and types of consumers in your marketing area. Knowing the number of prospects to receive your message is essential in planning and budgeting your further campaign. Knowing their characteristics, particularly the loyalty learning items described in the preceding chapter, is essential for designing, developing, and delivering the loyalty offer, and for completing the Loyalty Marketing Wheel.

Designing Transaction and Relationship Offers

The offers you manage can include three types of value that you use to make the offers irresistible to consumers:

- **Natural value** = benefits/costs that you have nothing to do with delivering but that consumers will gain automatically if they take up your offer. The natural health benefits of quitting smoking are an example, as are the built-in continuity and familiarity benefits of loyalty.
- **Current value** = benefits/costs that you have already included in your offer and that represent significant but not quite sufficient total value (when coupled with natural value) to win the consumers you are targeting—so you are improving the offer. This does not apply, of course, to an entirely new offer.
- **Added value** = benefits/costs that you consciously put into your offer to make it irresistible to targeted consumers. If yours is a new offer, it will include only added and natural value; if you are improving an existing offer, it can include all three categories.

The management tasks do not apply to all three categories of value. Natural benefits, for instance, occur regardless of whose offer the consumer takes, and you cannot add to them. Any natural value you can identify and make a strong case for, however, belongs in your communications, tracking, and reminding efforts. Similarly, existing benefits and costs are not subject to additional management effort unless they need to be improved, in which case they become added-value items. As with natural value, existing value belongs in your offer, but only for your communications, tracking, and reminding efforts.

The management step focuses on designing, developing, and delivering irresistible new or improved value. Both natural and existing value are important to management, however, as a basis for deciding the amount of added value that needs to be managed into the offer in order to make it irresistible. In rare circumstances, where consumer prospects are truly unaware of the original value or have little confidence in it, communications alone may suffice to convert consumers—and additional management effort is not necessary.

Normally, however, the management team is challenged to combine any natural and existing value already in the offer with value-adding changes or initiatives to make the offer one that consumers will not refuse. Arriving at the right combination is a challenge to both effectiveness and efficiency. Management must design, develop and deliver an offer that is sufficient to convert consumers to trial customers and eventually to loyal customers—but the offer must be realistic, not outrageously good or expensive.

Ideally, you will have learned that enough consumers can be converted if you add only *one* value or if you make *one* change in structure, process, or outcome that delivers multiple values. In chapter 1, building in a method of immediate relief of anxiety might have been the single offer improvement needed. In a weight management program, the single new or improved outcome of lasting weight loss could deliver multiple benefits to consumers: improved appearance, self-esteem, confidence in health and longevity, and improved sports performance, for example.[4]

An unfortunate tendency in many marketing efforts is to employ a shotgun approach to the design, development, and delivery of an offer: throw in everything *including* the proverbial kitchen sink and hope that it will be enough. Such an approach threatens the efficiency of offer management and the ability of the organization to gain value in return. You can use the learning process to develop a rifle approach instead, focusing on one or two highly significant value improvements or initiatives rather than on many insignificant ones. The learning process can also help identify an extended benefit well beyond that of the competition, for instance, including hotel, meals, and transportation arrangements for patients coming from out of town for care.

You have three categories of the marketing mix to work with in your management tasks:

- **Product value** = offering new or increased benefits to consumers.
- **Place value** = making it easier for consumers to gain those benefits.
- **Price value** = reducing the monetary costs, risks, time costs, and any other negative effects that taking your offer entails.

You may work on any one of them or on a mix of all three to design an irresistible and deliverable offer.

As the preceding chapter indicated, the marketing approach to the management of an offer entails the design of a unique or superior "value proposition" that tells consumer prospects: "If you become/remain our patient/member, you will enjoy more/better/sooner (particular benefits at better costs) . . . than you will get from any competing offer." In many cases, the design process can begin with such a proposition or even with a draft advertisement for the offer. If an irresistible value proposition can be created by the marketing communications staff, then management may figure out a way to deliver it.

By clarifying and focusing on a unique or superior value offer, you have the widest range of choices in managing tasks. (On the other hand, if learning has failed to identify the key values involved, you will be only guessing.) Even though management can translate a value proposition into reality, the effort works best when that value proposition, rather than an early presumption about the structure and process factors, is the explicit focus of your efforts. The best structure or process factor may be chosen by chance alone, but relying on chance is unnecessary and certainly risky.

With a clear value proposition in mind, managers can first investigate ways that will best deliver that value. In selecting the best approach, they can sense the feasibility and efficiency of the value and its best positioning in terms of overall operations and strategy. They can concept-test ideas and pilot-trial offers to see if consumers find the offer irresistible. Pilot testing can help if management wants to select the most effective and efficient option among competing delivery methods.

In general, offering a unique or superior benefit is the most powerful approach to making an offer irresistible. A unique benefit is stronger than a superior one, but if an offer is outstanding compared to rival offers, then it's close to being as good. Similarly, durable value is normally stronger than "during" value in attracting converts. Healthcare is uniquely positioned to make the biggest, longest-lasting differences to a consumer's quality of life. By delivering more value of the enduring kind, you can gain over rivals with offers at less enduring value.

By no means, however, can you ignore the "during" dimensions of healthcare encounters and relationships. No health organization's work is so valuable that its level of service quality and bedside manner makes no difference. Many progressive providers gain an enormous advantage when they choose to do something about the "during" value of their encounters with patients. Many of my clients have enjoyed dramatic improvements in their marketing and financial performance just by doing *something* more than their rivals to make encounters more pleasant, less costly, and more convenient for patients.

Health plans have a unique opportunity to compete in offering value. The quality of life value that patients and plan members gain may be worth far more to them than the costs imposed. Pregnant women appear to value ultrasound screening so much that they demand it even when there is no medical indication for it, and most would pay the charge out-of-pocket if they had to.[5] Similarly, men are demanding the new impotence drugs despite their high price and are expressing willingness to pay for some or all of the cost. Yet some health plans argue that such services should not be covered because they *only* enhance quality of life.[6] This may make management sense to some, but denying coverage for treatment because it has *only* a quality of life benefit has terrible marketing disadvantages.

Next comes the unique or superior ease of receiving the benefit, perhaps at home or at work, for example, rather than on site of the plan or provider. "Place" improvements can reduce the costs of time and stress for the consumer, for example, and often can be more important than dollar price reductions. Each place, convenience, or access factor under consideration should be examined in light of its benefit enhancement or cost reduction effect, with the particular benefit clearly identified and emphasized as the *end* of the effort, and the innovations and changes in hours, location, rules, or other factors as the *means* to that end.

The least useful offer dimension to consider is dollar price. First, a reduction in your price makes your revenue less, even if it does attract more consumers. You will have to attract a certain number of additional consumers just to make up for the loss in revenue. Second, for many offers a lower price hints, at least, at poorer quality. Consumers intrigued by lower insurance premiums, for example, may wonder what they will lose with the "budget"-priced health plan. Third, cutting your price typically will force you to actually reduce your quality, making the retention and future attraction of consumers problematic. Finally, price is the easiest thing in the world for your rivals to match or beat; it takes only the stroke of a pen.

Other "prices" you can reduce include the time, hassle, and stress costs that you may impose without intending to do so, and of which you may not even be aware. By gathering the right insights from prospects and loyal customers, you can identify those elements in your operation that produce costs to consumers without producing any benefit to you: these should be the earliest targets for elimination. Any negative aspect of your relationship with consumers can be targeted for price reduction and, in many cases, the effect can be promised in positive terms as money or time they can spend on something else.

Because each Medicare enrollee in an HMO costs anywhere from $500 to $1,500 to acquire, for example, their retention is essential to profitable plan performance. Yet cutting costs due to reduced prices can lead to reductions in service and to unhappy consumers. One survey found that 26 percent of interested prospect callers to an HMO's member service line had to leave voice messages, 48 percent did not receive the information or materials they requested within four weeks, and only 14 percent received follow-up calls. Cost-cutting in this case destroyed the positive effect of lower prices.[7]

In many markets, competition is forcing prices toward a uniform level or one with barely distinguishable differences, and the only way providers and plans can compete is on "quality" or benefit to consumers (and perhaps "convenience" or saved time and stress as well). The same phenomenon has already appeared among large retailers. The survivors will be those offering superior value of some kind.[8]

Although mainly a communications challenge, management may arrive at a point where offering unique or superior *confidence* in value becomes a competitive distinction, in addition to or as opposed to unique or superior value itself.[9] Making healthcare provider and plan choices is a risky business for consumers, and one where they are rarely able to make a trial purchase to check out value. Often they cannot tell for years if they got an effective treatment or chose a good plan, and some treatments can be judged with confidence only when they fail—for instance, preventive services.

If you can heighten consumer confidence in your offer over rival offers, particularly if the offers are all roughly equal in value, you should win a far larger share than the $1/n$ expected when n indistinguishable offers compete.[10] The comparative size of the larger share will depend on the level of greater confidence you can impart to consumers, and its duration. Although most of the methods for instilling confidence depend on communications rather than management, at least two ways exist in which management effort significantly affects consumer confidence.

First is the extent to which you are delivering consistent value at this time. Consistency of value promotes satisfaction among current customers and stimulates word-of-mouth "advertising" that should enhance consumer confidence in your new and improved offers. If your advertised value has consistently in fact, been delivered, your future advertising becomes more credible and thus more effective in promoting consumer confidence. As consumers try your new or improved offer, and gain the value they expected and desired (with perhaps a pleasant surprise or two as well), their confidence in gaining equal or better value in subsequent contacts is bound to grow.

The impact of past value delivery reliability on consumer confidence can be enhanced even further with a guarantee of value. In fact, this may be the only option when you or your offer, or both, lack a prior history with your consumer prospects. Management is involved because a true guarantee includes a stated manner of making up for any failures, and in most cases this will cost money. A guarantee to serve each patient in the ER within 15 minutes, or of patient satisfaction with each clinic visit, will cost whatever money-back or specified dollar recompense is included in the guarantee, as well as any added costs of minimizing failures to meet the guaranteed standard.

Not only will this come out of management's budget, in most cases, but any value delivery failures can cut into the net revenue for the department or organization affected. Management will be held responsible for minimizing such failures, lest the marketing effect of the guarantee be destroyed by service failures. Such failures will undermine both the financial success of the offer and the credibility of future communications. Guarantees rarely are sufficient to truly make up for not getting the promised value; but they make the promise more credible. If consumers' experience and subsequent word of mouth describe too many "horror tales" of promised value not received, the effect of the guarantee will disappear.

Designing the value offer begins with being precise in specifying the value(s) you will include in a new offer or will add to a current one. These can include any one of the following or any mix:

- improved health, feeling good, pride in accomplishment, and so on, via health promotion services and risk reduction programs;
- reduced risk and incidence of preventable disease and injury;
- avoided time costs, hassles, and out-of-pocket payments thanks to self-care manuals, triage, and training;
- avoided chronic disease crises and complications, with their medical care utilization and costs, and their disruptions in normal activities—and perhaps, as a result, a continuation of treasured independence—due to disease management programs;
- cures, restoration of function, and recovery from a wide range of diseases and injuries, including the financial and career benefits gained;
- rehabilitation and an improved ability to cope with conditions from which recovery is limited, including the financial and career benefits gained; and
- an acceptable, even admirable end of life, including its impact on family and friends.

In addition to these durable and healthcare-focused kinds of value, the offer can be designed to add "during" and non-healthcare benefits. You can emphasize small gestures of good personal service, in contrast to the increasingly depersonalized services consumers receive from ATMs and computerized phone find-it-yourself systems.[11] Your offers of educational, health promotion, support group, and similar programs can include socializing opportunities, that add to their medical value.[12]

Your knowledge about loyalty and your own expertise should indicate which of these benefits or other "during" benefits will prove irresistible to targeted consumers—and are feasible to deliver at a profit. In general, whether ideas for value design come from consumers themselves, from your own staff, or from a combination of the two, you should validate the design with consumers before you go further. An HMO that "improved" its services via an electronic ID card system costing over $300,000 discovered too late that the system provided no value that consumers wanted.[13]

Such a mistake can be averted by including targeted consumers in the design process.[14] Using ongoing consumer input and feedback in planning new or improved offers can prevent the more egregiously misguided designs and avoid subsequent wasted effort and expense. Concept and pilot testing can do the same. Getting consumer comments not only on the value(s) you intend to deliver, but also on the specific structures and processes you intend to use in doing so, will provide the most practical input.

Building in consumer choice is another way of dealing with the unpredictability, changeability, and variability of consumer preferences. Enough choices can allow consumers to tailor particular experiences and relationships to their individual wishes. In addition, choice delivers value of its own by increasing consumers' control over their world.[15] Consumers have shown a willingness to pay up to $20 per month more in premiums, for example, in order to have their own choice of provider.[16]

A special challenge in designing value offers faces those health plans and providers at capitation risk. Unfortunately, but in fact, consumers who are sickest stand to gain the greatest value from plans and providers both. Consumers with chronic conditions and those with major acute injuries and illnesses can gain dramatically in the quality and quantity of their lives through health services covered by plans. As a result, plans and providers who do particularly well at delivering value stand both to retain more loyal sick consumers and, by reputation, to gain more of them among their new recruits.

By contrast, basically healthy consumers may have little or no contact with plans and providers. What value do they gain that can promote their loyalty or attract more of their healthy peers? Although all consumers may feel some benefit thanks to the security of knowing that insurance and providers are standing by in case of need, that benefit is uniformly available in all plans and providers so it offers no competitive advantage or reason for continued loyalty to one over another.

Plans and providers at risk are both ethically and legally bound to deliver value to sicker, higher-cost consumers, but by delivering such value they risk the anti-selection dilemma.[17] The best way to counter this is through offering and delivering such value to healthy consumers that the risk is balanced, if not outweighed, by pro-selection and retention among the healthy. In most cases this will mean using health promotion, risk reduction, prevention, early detection, and self-care programs to add to the quality of healthy lives—not merely to reduce demand.[18]

Both plans and providers can promote consumer loyalty by multiplying the contacts and the benefit-adding opportunities they offer consumers. Of particular value is information. Sending out useful, understandable information that means something to individual consumers is one of the simplest and least expensive ways to deliver added value and to promote contacts with infrequent customers. Enabling consumers to gain information on their own can be even more beneficial as they will look for the precise information of interest at the exact time of their interest.

It is easy to grant loyal consumers perks such as access to the health library, invitations to health education seminars, and contact with disease and grief support groups. Newsletters can be customized to particular consumer interests. Call centers can provide ongoing access to information, enabling consumers to make more informed decisions, reduce costs, and add to their quality of life. Internet access to Web sites and chat rooms not only enables consumers to gain information; it supplies an indirect measure of values important to them, thus enhancing your own loyalty learning.

Although it almost always makes good sense to validate consumer preferences and to check on the value you intend to deliver, some benefits are fairly safe to design into an offer even if no consumers have mentioned them. Saving time, either because you deliver the value sooner (e.g., lab test results) or deliver a service more promptly, should be perceived as a benefit by most consumers. They will usually welcome reductions in the hassle and stress experienced in undergoing service processes—completing paperwork, having to repeat the same information over and over, or having difficulty parking. If a major investment is required to deliver such benefits, however, it is a good idea to validate their worth.

Developing the Offer

However well designed, the offer at some point must be translated into reality. Management must acquire, organize, direct, and control the resources needed to deliver the designed value (or something close enough to it). And this must be done in ways that are economically feasible and that permit you to make the offer at a price that attracts consumers and yields a decent return. Your organization must develop and maintain an information system that facilitates the customized delivery of the most attractive and satisfying value to the individual consumer.[19]

While most of the development process depends on the particulars of the organization, the offer, and the targeted consumers, a few general recommendations on that process can perhaps ensure successful communication and delivery. The first recommendation is to include in the delivery system some means of enabling the consumer to gain the *most value* available from the offer. It's always good to build in more versus less personal contact—to provide enough information to enable novice consumers to match veterans in gaining benefit as inexpensively as possible.

It is essential to hire *capable staff* who are oriented to the delivery of your designed values. Consumers themselves can help in the selection and orientation of staff. Hiring and training staff especially for the consumers you are pursuing can help; one HMO was able to reduce its Medicare turnover rate by 75 percent this way.[20] Humana hired an entire staff of people to make early and frequent contacts with new Medicare enrollees and got similar results.[21]

Organizing for retention can also help. Many hospitals have organized staff based on their markets and consumer segments, in contrast to the traditional focus on functions or service lines.[22] In its pursuit of loyalty, MedNet HMO of Cleveland, Ohio created an enrollee retention department to educate members and answer their questions.[23]

The main thrust of these recommendations is that you invest time, effort, and resources specifically in pursuit of retention and loyalty as opposed to a focus solely on the "conquest" of consumers by competing to recruit the most.[24]

Upon selecting, training, organizing, and orienting quality employees, it also helps to gear their performance objectives and their rating and reward systems to the delivery of value. At a minimum their work can be evaluated based on the levels of consumer loyalty as well as the satisfaction ratings they achieve. Ideally, personnel efforts will be assessed based on the value that these people *deliver to consumers*, not just the value they gain in return. Individual employees responsible for delivering value will be rewarded along with their managers and executives, whose contributions may have been less direct. This approach has been used by American Express in rewarding its account representatives based on the amount their merchant clients gained.[25] Medline rewards its medical supplies sales representatives who enable customers to save money by arranging retroactively for those reps to share in the savings.[26]

Finally, you should retain these employees themselves and earn their loyalty. Although people can be somewhat loyal to abstractions such as brands and organizations, it is hard to overstate the personal foundations for most forms of loyalty. Customers of mutual fund firms have left en masse when the fund manager has gone elsewhere, for example; physicians hired by hospitals usually take their patients with them if they leave; and patients have defected in droves from HMOs when the provider network has dropped their personal physicians.

Employee satisfaction and loyalty have been shown to be two of the best predictors of customer satisfaction and loyalty. One survey, for example, found that a 10 percent reduction in employee turnover led to 1–3 percent increases in customer retention—and a 5 percent increase in customer retention led to 25–125 percent increases in profits.[26] When employees consider themselves champions of customers, and customers view them the same way, the satisfaction and retention of both likely increases.[27]

Value Delivery

Even with excellent design and systems development, value delivery depends on the day-to-day behavior of the individuals who enable consumers to gain specific benefits and minimize their costs. A number of excellent works available on service management and marketing (some of which are listed at the end of this chapter) will help you improve daily contacts. Two general recommendations can be made, however: the empowerment of staff to deliver the best value experience and of consumers to receive it—in every encounter.[28]

Picker-Commonwealth, for example, found that one of the greatest service failures in hospitals was the inadequate preparation of discharged patients for what would happen next: a lack of necessary patient empowerment to maximize their own recovery and, if possible, to prevent recurrence of the problem. Only 55 percent of discharged patients reported getting help with the transition back home, and 20 percent reported encountering "serious problems" in that regard.[29] In research conducted regularly when I was CMO of Provenant Health Partners in Denver, Colorado, a measure that rated discharge experience was the most powerful predictor of patient loyalty six months later.

Consumer empowerment at discharge and follow-up contacts after discharge demonstrate the kind of long-term interest in patients that promotes loyalty. Such interest also can alleviate patients' anxiety over symptoms and reassure them when they have questions.[30] An ability to *anticipate* likely patient problems and concerns—which experienced providers certainly should have—can be among the most powerful promoters of satisfaction and loyalty.[31]

The reduction of anxiety should be a focus of interactions with patients and enrollees at every encounter.[32] Anxiety over one's health or symptoms drives most of a person's contacts with providers; anxiety over coverage, claims handling, and bill paying drives a substantial proportion of personal contacts with health plans. Staff should be trained to sense anxiety and to alleviate it. Consumers should feel relieved that they contacted your organization and rate it the best source of help they know.

Empowering employees is the only way to handle well the idiosyncratic needs and wants of consumers and the unpredictable problems and service failures that are sure to occur. You should authorize individual staff to *demonstrate* their understanding and concern about the consumers with whom they interact and their knowledge of the best answers to individual consumers problems and concerns.[33] Providers need to identify precisely the relationship and decision-making process each patient desires *at each encounter* and should arrange to play their parts accordingly.[34]

Although loyalty and enduring value are the chief aims of loyalty marketing, keep in mind that satisfaction with individual encounters and the "during" value that each can deliver are essential contributors to these ends.[35] Successful responses to the emotional dimensions of most encounters are key.[36] Personal gestures that individualize the encounter— going an extra mile (or at least a few yards) to address specific needs and requests—can make an enormous difference.[37] Small acts of kindness such as smiling, using the consumer's preferred form of address, and offering encouragement and reassurance can be critical to "during" value.[38]

Just as involving employees in loyalty learning promotes their enthusiasm in carrying out the overall marketing initiative, so too does including them in discussions of the design, development, and delivery of a potentially irresistible marketing offer help ensure their cooperation in its delivery. Including or not including decision makers in addition to line employees in these sessions is a judgment call, depending on the importance and probability of their support without such participation, and on whether they will add to the quality of your offer development or impose ideas that will steer you away from the best offer.

Connections

Clearly one chapter cannot cover the decades of findings published in the literature, nor can it incorporate all of my own personal experience in managing value. But through the brief summary of key points in this chapter, my intent is to place the management of value in the context of loyalty marketing and to clarify the connections between the management step and other steps in the value delivery chain.

Loyalty learning feeds forward into the management step the information needed, for example, to choose the right loyalty targets and to design, develop, and deliver the irresistible value offer. But management also feeds back to the learning step those things that consumers say and do during particular encounters and interactions, and the observations of employees. Through identifying the value that is ultimately to be delivered, management gives the promise communication step its direction on what to say, the tracking step its briefing on what to measure, and the reminding step its instructions on what to remind consumers about.

The more you appreciate the role of management in loyalty marketing, and its contributions to the other stakeholder roles as well as its gains from them, the more effectively and efficiently you will be able to move the wheel to achieve the results and return on investment you are after. The connections among the elements of the wheel will be emphasized, perhaps belabored, through the next chapters.

Figure 2-2 Management Connections

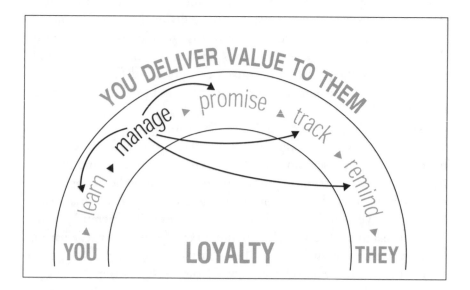

Action Recommendations

✓ Identify the sets of consumer targets for your unique loyalty proposition, including current customers and prospects as appropriate. _____

✓ Design the specific loyalty value offer you will make and deliver to them, based on your loyalty learning from chapter 1, by combining natural, current, and added value, in both the during and the enduring categories, as needed. _____

✓ Combine product, place, and price elements in specifics of the offer, and pretest the offer with targeted consumers using concept or pilot tests, as appropriate. _____

✓ Adjust the offer design based on consumer responses together with your own internal capabilities and limitations. _____

✓ Arrive at a specific loyalty offer that is unique or superior compared to rivals' offers and that you can deliver consistently to consumer customers—or at least arrive at an offer for which you can promote unique or superior levels of confidence among consumers. _____

✓ Acquire and organize the resources you will need to deliver that loyalty offer consistently and profitably. _____

✓ Direct and ensure the consistent delivery of your offer to your consumer customers, with continuous value improvement where feasible. _____

✓ Devise and employ performance evaluation and reward structures based on your employees' success in delivering value to your consumer customers, to be tied to your value delivery tracking system (chapter 4). _____

References

1. Anderson, D. 1982. "The Satisfied Customer: Service Return Behavior in the Obstetric Market." *Journal of Health Care Marketing* 2, no. 4 (fall): 25–33.

2. Bell, C. 1994. *Customers as Partners: Building Relationships That Last.* San Francisco: Berrett-Koehler.

3. "Analysis Looks at Member Strategy for Health Benefit Plans." *Healthcare Strategy Alert* (January 1998): 8.

4. Myers, J. 1996. *Segmentation and Positioning for Strategic Marketing Decisions.* Chicago: American Marketing Association.

5. Beck, C., et al. 1997. *Partnership for Health: Building Relationships Between Women and Health Caregivers.* Mahwah, NJ: Lawrence Erlbaum.

6. Hilzenrath, D. 1998. "Kaiser Will Halt Viagra Coverage." *Denver Post* (20 June): 1A, 21A.

7. Clark, B. 1998. "Older, Sicker, Smarter and Redefining Quality: The Older Consumer's Quest for Patient-Driven Service." *Healthcare Forum Journal* 41, no. 1 (January/February): 26–30.

8. Berry, L. 1996. "Retailers with a Future." *Marketing Management* 5, no. 1 (spring): 38–46.

9. MacStravic, S. 1998. "Marketing by Means of the Confidence Factor." *Health Care Strategic Management* 16, no. 1 (January): 1, 19–23.

10. Marder, E. 1996. *The Laws of Choice: Predicting Customer Behavior.* New York: Free Press.

11. Braus, P. 1997. *Marketing Health Care to Women.* Ithaca, NY: American Demographics.

12. Cross, R., and J. Smith. 1997. "The Customer Value Chain." *Marketing Tools* (January/February): 14–18.

13. Iacobucci, D. 1996. "The Quality Improvement Customers Didn't Want." *Harvard Business Review* 74, no. 1 (January/February): 20–36.

14. Peeno, L. 1998. "What Is the Value of a Voice?" *US News & World Report* (9 March): 40–46.

15. Miller, D. 1998. "How Marketers Can Build Support for Brand Development." *Strategic Health Care Marketing* 15 (10 October): 4–6.

16. MacStravic, S. 1996. "The Disease Management Dilemma." *Health Care Strategic Management* 14, no. 6 (June): 18–19.

17. ———. 1997. " 'Managing' Demand: The Wrong Paradigm." *Managed Care Quarterly* 5, no. 4 (autumn): 8–17.

18. Herreria, J. 1997. "One-to-One Approach Catches On." *Profiles in Healthcare Marketing* 13, no. 5 (September/October): 5–8.

19. "Customer Loyalty Initiatives in Action." *Healthcare Strategy Alert* (January 1998): 6–8.

20. "Currents: Spending on Saving." *Hospitals & Health Networks* (5 July 1997): 12.

21. Flory, J. 1995. "CEO Takes Creative Approach to Manage Change." *Strategic Health Care Marketing* 12, no. 8 (August): 8–9.

22. Dempsey, W. S., and S. Mendel. 1994. "It's No Longer Words and Music: Marketing in a Capitated Environment." *Group Practice Journal* 43, no. 3 (May/June): 46–51.

23. "Finders Keepers: Marketing Metrics Show More Firms Are Using Retention Marketing Tactics." *Marketing Tools* (March/April 1995): 30–31.

24. Whiteley, R., and D. Hessan. 1996. *Customer Centered Growth.* Reading, MA: Addison-Wesley.

25. "Services Marketing: Lessons Learned From the Best." *Services Marketing Today* 12, no. 6 (December 1996): 1, 5.

26. Bell, C., and R. Zemke. 1992. *Managing Knock Your Socks Off Service.* New York: AMACOM.

27. Zimmerman, D., et al. 1996. *The Health Care Customer Service Revolution.* Chicago: Irwin Professional.

28. Webster, F. 1994. "Defining the New Marketing Concept." *Marketing Management* 1 (4): 22–31.

29. Gerteis, M. 1993. "What Patients Really Want." *Health Management Quarterly* 15, no. 3 (third quarter): 2–6.

30. Byerly, L. 1996. "How Patients Define 'Service'. " *Health Progress* 77, no. 4 (July/August): 96–98.

31. Greco, S. 1995. "The Road to One to One Marketing." *INC.* 17 (14 October): 56–66.

32. Dunn, E. et al. 1995. "Decreasing Anxiety." *Journal of Health Care Marketing* 15, no. 1 (spring): 21–23.

33. Bernstein, A., and D. Freiermuth. 1988. *The Health Professional's Marketing Handbook.* Chicago: Year Book Medical.

34. Eggar, R. 1978. "I Make My Patients Be Their Own Doctors." *Medical Economics* 55 (12 June): 82–90.

35. "Can't Get No Customer Satisfaction?" *Quality Digest* 16, no. 8 (August 1996): 13–14.

36. Dubé, L., M-C. Bélanger, and E. Trudeau. 1996. "The Role of Emotions in Health Care Satisfaction." *Journal of Health Care Marketing* 16, no. 2 (summer): 45–51.

PROMISING VALUE

Figure 3-1

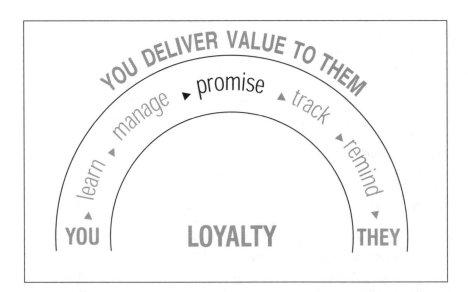

"PROMISING" VALUE does not mean literally to *promise* specific benefits and costs to consumers. The intent is to create in their minds confident *expectations* that they will gain unique or superior value by doing business with you or, at least, unique or superior *confidence* that they will gain from you the value they seek as compared to their level of confidence in rival offers. On the other hand, in looking for loyalty from consumers, it is wise to "promise" value as if you really mean it—to communicate only that value you are sure you will deliver, given the success of your management in identifying, planning, and arranging for value delivery.

This chapter does not describe the full range of possibilities and techniques of the trade in marketing communications. Far more than one book would be needed for such a task. Rather, it discusses your options regarding the identification and numbering of benefits to promise and the ways in which you can deal with costs to make an accurate, irresistible promise of value. The promise of value is key to the *beginning* of the loyalty building process among targeted consumers. In this chapter, I specifically address the wisdom and timing of promises to deliver value as well as the variety of ways to communicate value, from vague suggestions to outright guarantees.

Identifying the Value to Promise

In the learning process you have identified a range of benefits (and costs), and you have arranged to deliver them in the management process. Now it's time to make choices regarding which benefits to promise. With the consumer's satisfaction, delight, and long-term loyalty in mind, you do not want to promise benefits that you are unsure will be delivered to them and perceived by them as beneficial. Quite apart from any legal risk of misleading, defrauding, or deceiving people in your communications, it is a waste of energy to try to produce loyalty by promising value that will not be delivered and perceived as value.

On the other hand, you have to promise enough value to entice consumers to try your offer for the first time. One of the "art versus science" dimensions of marketing lies in balancing the need to entice consumers with the desire to delight and retain them. A higher level of success in enticing consumers is possible if you promise greater value than you will deliver, but you will draw greater delight and retention success by delivering more value than you promised. How much value is enough to promise for the enticement effect, yet allows room for a pleasant surprise or two for the loyalty effect? That question is answerable only through an understanding of your consumer prospects and some experience in promising and delivering value to them.

On the cost side of the promising value challenge, it is wise to describe every cost that consumers are likely to experience, because a negative surprise—that is, any aspect of the actual delivery experience that is worse than expected—obviously will produce dissatisfaction. In addition to the costs consciously built into your offer to provide revenue, efficiency, or other performance values to your organization, you should identify and communicate costs that consumers will tell you about when they describe their "during" and enduring experiences in practice.

If you have designed and delivered the consumer experience in a way that creates uncertainty, stress, and wasted time, money, and effort for consumers, you have two choices. The first is to reconsider your offer design and delivery to eliminate such costs, particularly those that yield no value to you; or, second, you can include those costs whenever you communicate promised value in order to inoculate consumers against unpleasant surprises. Generally, removing the costs is best, although, in some cases, doing so may cost you more than it is worth in enhancing value to consumers.

In promising benefits, by contrast, you can deliberately hold some in reserve and not include them in your promises of value. Some may be omitted because you are not sure enough that you will deliver them to all consumers, or that all prospects would perceive them as benefits in any case. These "reserves" may be used as pleasant contingent surprises: do your best to deliver them; track to check on your success with them; and, finally, remind consumers of them to generate the perception of an unexpected but welcome benefit. You can reserve many benefits, including some you are sure you will deliver, if you don't need them to make your promise of value irresistible.

Such an approach has particular advantages when you are promising value to consumers who vary widely in their desires and expectations for value. So long as enough consumers find the promises of core benefits sufficiently enticing, you can reserve the indirect benefits until you have captured the prospects' interest. You may promise only weight loss, for example, to consumers interested in a range of indirect benefits, from sports performance improvement to better health to more energy to improved appearance. If you decide to promise only the loss of weight, you can arrange to track and remind individual consumers of the specific indirect benefit they most wish for—after you have determined what that benefit is.

Including all of the probable benefits in your promises of value can enhance the success of marketing communications in attracting consumers, but it may undermine the effect on long-term loyalty. Even if all of the value promised is delivered, no room will be left for pleasant surprises because you will have delivered only what you promised. This also means that you will not be able to consciously add benefits for loyal consumers:

they will receive exactly the same benefits as the first-time converts and no more.

Having some pleasant surprises in store at the outset helps to promote initial delight as opposed to mere satisfaction. Reserving some potential benefits for future delivery helps in delivering some repeat pleasant surprises for long-term loyal consumers. Here again, only marketing information and experience with particular consumers will suggest which of the benefits to include in promises, which to reserve for pleasant surprises for first-time customers, and which to reserve for long-term customers as later special perks or surprises.

The main thing is to consciously decide on the benefits to use and the ones to reserve, rather than to lump them all into your initial offer. If you underestimate the benefits to include in your initial offer, you can always adjust your promised value upward to achieve the enticement success you are after. If you overdo the initial offer, leaving nothing for a surprise, however, you cannot go back and reduce the offer without losing credibility: you will be promoting deselection among past customers if you reduce your promise of value, and dissatisfaction among repeat customers if you reduce the actual value delivered.

Categories of Benefits

You can include three categories of benefits in your promises: "natural," current, and added. *Natural benefits* are the improvements that naturally arise from a particular consumer behavior; they would enjoy these benefits from any provider or plan. The positive health effects of quitting cigarettes are examples, as are the potential effects of losing weight. These may be powerful reasons for consumers to choose to sign up with a smoking cessation or weight loss program, but they are not reasons for preferring one provider or plan over another.

This does not make these benefits lower in importance than other categories of benefits, however. If you are the first to mention such benefits, while rivals do not even offer the programs, you can gain many converts. If you cite your success in achieving both weight loss and the indirect benefits of losing pounds while your rivals cite only weight loss per se, you can gain so long as your success in weight loss per se is competitive. If you cite reports from past customers that bolster the prospects' greater confidence that they can achieve specific benefits, you may gain versus rivals who mention only the potential of the benefits.

Where the natural benefits of your promised outcomes are the most important reasons for consumers to prefer one program over another, then it is likely to be consumer confidence in gaining those benefits that will tell. By measuring the benefits that past consumers have actually achieved and by publishing these measures as results of your program, you may gain simply by being explicit about your program's success and its benefits to consumers, while your rivals are not, relying instead on the benefits implied in consumers' expectations of program outcomes.

Current benefits are those already available in your past offer and already being enjoyed by your customers. Like natural benefits, these may be as important as any in converting prospects. Some consumers may not be aware of such benefits or simply may have forgotten them. You may be able to gain converts merely by making prospects more confident of receiving the benefits you have always delivered. At a minimum, combining your current benefits with any natural or added benefits can make your offer more powerful than focusing on new benefits alone.

Added benefits are those that are new as far as consumers are concerned. These can be the most challenging to promise since you will have no track record to rely on. Your past customers will not have spread their enthusiasm about these benefits because you've never offered or delivered them. You have no statistics or case histories to cite, no testimonials to use. If your credibility is low because you are new in the market or have not established a trusting relationship with consumers, added value will be the most difficult category of benefits to promise; yet it's the category where creating positive expectation may have the greatest impact on converting prospects.

"During" Benefits versus Durable Benefits

Each of the natural, current, and added benefits may fall into either, or both, the "during" or durable dimension of value. The most commonly promised benefits in services marketing are of the during variety, benefits that occur only during the service experience itself and are perceived only at that time. You may promise, for instance, that patients will feel welcome, and will save time, thanks to your brief wait or speedy screening process. You may promise that the person who answers the member service phone will answer plan members' questions, or that on-site screening or enrollment services will enable the member to avoid the need to travel.

Not to belittle these benefits, but healthcare has the potential for making dramatic positive differences that last a lifetime! By and large, promises of lasting benefit are likely to be more attractive than are promises of immediate but transitory gains. The cosmetic surgeon who can promise more gradual aging and the psychological benefits of an improved appearance is likely to attract more patients than the one who promises only prompt service. The health plan that promises improved health or better management of chronic disease will do better than the plan promising only easy enrollment.

The difference between "during" and durable benefits is clearly one of degree rather than kind. Patients may take away from their healthcare encounter an overall good feeling that lasts for hours or days after the visit. A plan member may gain not only the relief from anxiety provided by a phone triage service, but information as well on self-care or child care that instills in the caller a general sense of confidence in handling future concerns. The challenge is to promise the duration as well as the nature of the benefits you'll deliver, and the longer the better, provided your promise is accurate.

Explicit Benefits Versus Implicit Benefits

Another choice in the promising process involves whether or not to be explicit about benefits, costs, and value. Traditional marketing communications frequently describe structural features, process events, or attributes of both, with the hope, at least, that consumers will make the connection between these more easily manageable elements and the outcomes and benefits that make them worthwhile. If consumers do make the right connection consistently, then an explicit benefit promise may be superfluous.

On the other hand, mentioning the features, events, and attributes only of structure and process may lead to consumer misunderstanding about the significance of features and events or the meaning of attributes. Consumers may interpret implicit statements as having benefits implications that were not intended and will not result. Or they may lean toward rivals who make the benefits explicit, perhaps even promising or guaranteeing them, while you are promising only structure and process elements.

Explicit promises of benefits should be the more powerful approach in most cases, although it can be more legally risky if you do not deliver the promised value. And because you do not actually *deliver* the benefits, but only the experiences and outcomes that produce those benefits, your promise of explicit benefits necessarily adds risk. You face a typical trade-off dilemma where, in order to obtain the greater effect of your explicit promises, you must accept the added risk.

One example of the use of explicit benefits in communicating your value promise is the "qualifying approach," beginning with the explicit outcome or benefit you intend to deliver expressed in the communications headline or "grabber" and the grabber then used to gain the attention of precisely those whom you wish to attract. Examples could include, "Want to Lose Weight?," "Hoping for a Better Love Life?," or "Looking to Prevent Complications of Diabetes?" Such headlines could then lead into discussions of the ways in which your programs or services achieve that explicit outcome or value.

Findings Ways to Promise Value

The first thing to recognize in deciding how to promise value is that it is not your intentions that count: what counts is the consumer's interpretation of the message you are communicating. You may be able to argue logically that you never intended to promise, indeed did not imply, any promise of value. But if the inference is there and consumers act on that inference—and if they do not subsequently obtain the value they think you promised—you have disappointed them and you should expect to lose them as loyal customers. Moreover, if you are taken to court and charged with false and misleading advertising, the court's judgment of a reasonable inference from your communications—not your intention— will form the basis for the verdict.[1]

That said, you have available a clear variety of communications approaches to use, ranging widely in the degree of promising involved. The approaches to use depend both on the value you are promising and on the degree to which you intend to be accountable for your promise. Some examples will be presented in order of the degree of risk involved for the "promisor," from low to high. They correlate, as well, with the extent of likely impact on the "promisee."

Objective Description: The Least Risk

The safest approach to promising value is to describe objectively that which is true. This approach applies primarily to structure and process features and events that can be described in an objective manner, sure to be true for all consumers. Structural features are best, because they are true, independent of consumers, and are therefore verifiably true for all. Sponsorship/ownership, location, services offered, hours, and so on are safe to promise, and consumers may well translate them into value. You may promise events, such as the length of time for patients to wait or the time it will take to process a claim, as long as you are convinced that these events actually will transpire as described or will have only a slight negative impact from the few failures bound to occur.

It is equally possible to describe outcomes and benefits or costs in objective terms, for example, through the use of statistics. Citing the percentage of heart attack patients who survived in the most recent reporting period compared to the state's average survival rate for MIs is a practice used by Memorial Health Services in Long Beach, California.[2] The increasing use of "report cards" on healthcare providers and health plans poses a likelihood of growth in the use of outcomes data in advertising. This entails little risk, so long as the information is accurate, although your published outcomes data may become embarrassing if your organization's performance declines compared to that of your rivals.

Publishing information on the benefits delivered to past customers is less common, if only because measuring benefits to consumer quality of life is less common. As soon as a provider or health plan begins to collect data on clinical outcomes and perceived benefits delivered to consumers, it can easily publish the data as objective descriptions of its performance. The data can be compiled for the overall population served or for special population segments, such as women, children, seniors, minorities, and so forth, and published accordingly. The tracking of such data will be described in the next chapter.

You may be highly selective regarding the outcomes and benefit data you publish. Making public only the data that show your organization in a good, perhaps best, light can make you look good. There is risk, however, if you deliberately avoid mentioning data that will make you look bad or not as good, while you appear to imply that your published data are representative. Your credibility will actually be enhanced if you publish "two-sided" messages in which you include both good and bad data. Where you can cite excellent outcomes and benefits in areas of the greatest interest to consumers and mediocre outcomes and benefits in areas where fewer consumers care, the negative impact of admitting your weaknesses may be minimal.

Using your collected data on benefits in advertising can give you an advantage over rivals in situations where you are the first to publish such data. When rivals tout their excellence in terms of structures and processes, even outcomes, while you cite the benefits that your customers have reported, your reports may be more credible because they are based on consumer reports versus your own claims. And they may be more powerful in areas where your reports describe precisely the benefits consumers are after, while rival reports rely on a consumer interpretation of the same—but only implied—benefits.

When you describe the subjective attributes of your structures and processes, your pure description is not objective and may not be credible. Almost everyone will believe you if you cite objectively your location and the services you offer, for example, but if you claim that your location is convenient and your services comprehensive, the same believability may not apply. On the other hand, you may cite consumers' ratings of the convenience of your location and the comprehensiveness of your services to back up your claims, or you may simply rely on their ratings to persuade your prospects. Although the latter are still subjective judgments, the fact that they are the judgments of consumers, and are objectively reported, will make them more credible.

Indirect Suggestion: A Little Riskier

An increasingly common approach to promising value is the indirect suggestion rather than the objective description of the value you offer and deliver to consumers. This approach is virtually never used with objective structural features, but it may be used with process events. Rather than citing statistics on the number of callers answered by the third ring, the number of claims processed within 30 days, or the number of minutes spent on the average wait in your waiting room, you can suggest your performance via radio or TV demonstration.

Showing a call being answered politely on the second ring, and demonstrating the manner in which your member service representative or receptionist handles typical calls can suggest a variety of service attributes, from promptness to courtesy to efficiency.

The words in an advertising message are often carefully chosen to suggest and imply rather than to promise and make explicit what consumers can expect. For instance, "we are committed to . . . (some attribute, outcome, or benefit)" or "we will help you achieve . . . (some outcome or benefit)" are both statements commonly used to avoid actually promising anything. Using a picture, testimonial, or case history of a "typical" successful example is equally common. Legally speaking, any such example should be typical, in fact as well as in representation, or the communications may be deemed misleading and actionable. Practically speaking, the example had better be characteristic of what a consumer will experience, or you will be sacrificing loyalty to gain a few new shoppers.

One cosmetic surgery ad mentioned " . . . how profoundly appearances on the outside affect the way we feel about ourselves inside" alongside a smiling, attractive woman. Such a suggestive approach only hints at the natural benefits available from cosmetic surgery, neither promising anything specific nor claiming any unique or superior expertise. If this is meant to interest people in seeking cosmetic surgery, per se, such an approach makes sense, although it will not help providers in places where all of the potential demand is already being met and gaining a greater share of that demand is the aim.

One ad promises only that "we help keep you well"—another asserts that "our mission is to keep you happy." Such expressions are promises to exert effort toward a benefit; they don't promise the benefit per se. If consumers infer a promise of benefit, these suggestions may be enough, depending on how explicit rivals are in their promises. However many "weasel words" you use in communications, there is always a Catch-22. If your words are too indirect and noncommittal, you may influence your prospects only slightly while you remain safe; yet if you achieve confident expectations of the benefits you only hint at, and thereby gain many converts, you may be held liable for false and misleading advertising because of your promise impact.

Predictions Versus Promises: Riskier Still

Making a prediction while being perceived to be making a promise may be one of the most common and annoying types of miscommunication in everyone's business and personal daily life. It used to be that you could clearly differentiate between a prediction and a promise. If you were predicting what you would do, you would say: "I *shall* (do something)." A promise would be stated as "I *will* (do it)." If you intended to predict what another person would do or experience, you would say: "You *will* . . . (gain a benefit, for example)" —while if you promised such an outcome, you would say: "You *shall* . . . (get it)." If this grammatical usage were still common and understood, it would be possible to distinguish the intention. It appears, however, that this distinction is not being taught or learned today, and in any case, the distinction is easily hidden through using '*ll* rather than specifying shall or will.

If you intend to promise a benefit, it is probably best to do so explicitly, saying something like "We promise . . . ," or "We will be sure (to do something)," or "We will ensure that (you experience something)" rather than taking a chance on its possible interpretation as a mere prediction. Conversely, if you intend only to predict, make that clear as well: "We predict that most of you will (experience some benefit)," or "We intend to (do something)," so that consumers do not misinterpret your prediction as a promise.

Once your intentions are firmly decided, you should test whether your words are precise in conveying them. Pretesting copy of specific messages to learn their consumer interpretations can both protect you against harm if you intend only to predict a benefit, and promote greater effects if you intend to promise it. You can use the results of such pretests as evidence in court, if the test shows that consumers saw only a prediction.

Publishing or posting a Patient's or Member's Bill of Rights is a good way to communicate the benefits that consumers can expect from a provider or plan. The wording of this bill of rights may express predictions or promises or even suggestions:

Suggestion: "you have the right to expect . . . " (only says what consumers might expect, not what they will get); "we are committed to . . . "; "our plan is designed to . . . "
Prediction: "patients will get . . . "
Promise: "we will ensure that patients get . . . "
Guarantee: "patients will get . . . or their money back."

All of these approaches can enable the provider or plan to promote the benefits—the value—that prospects and loyal customers can expect. The approaches vary only in the extent to which they commit the organization to delivering such benefits, although the difference in terms of what consumers think they have been promised may be slight.

Specific statements of what patients have the right to expect can cover structural features, process events, outcomes, or benefits/limited costs. For plans these can include the right to specific service coverage, appeals of denials, or answers to questions within some time period, for instance. And patients may have the right to privacy and confidentiality, to play a role in making treatment decisions, to be listened to, to feel safe and comfortable, and to enjoy peace of mind (Baker, p. 37).[3]

Guarantees: Only If You're Sure You'll Deliver

A guarantee may seem even stronger than a promise and therefore may carry more risk. This may depend, however, on the wording of your guarantee. If you say simply that "we guarantee that you will (have some experience, gain some benefit)," consumers and the courts are likely to interpret that as an unconditional guarantee. Then, if the value—perhaps tens of thousands or even millions of dollars worth—is not delivered, consumers may well sue for that full value.

Conversely, if your guarantee is limited and specific (e.g., "we guarantee your satisfaction or your money back") both your consumers and the courts are likely to limit their interpretation to your promised recompense. Your liability in that case is limited to the recompense you promised. It becomes a penalty you absorb, rather than the total value of your guaranteed outcome or benefit. Kaiser Permanente has guaranteed satisfaction with clinic services to patients or it will pay them a $25 penalty.[4] Blue Cross/Blue Shield has promised patient satisfaction at its clinics in Ohio or it will write off the next month's premium payment.[5]

More expensive guarantees, of objective outcomes rather than satisfaction, have been made by fertility clinics. One promised that its clients would become pregnant or their money would be refunded (Baker, p. 160)[3]; another promised delivery of a baby or money back.[6] Clearly, the latter would be a more powerful competitive guarantee, since it relates to what consumers are really after, not just getting pregnant, but having a baby. While this is not a guarantee of benefit per se, it is about as close as you can get with an objective clinical outcome.

If you intend to make an accountable promise, for which you can be sued for the full value of the promised experience, outcome, or benefit, by all means make that promise explicit, and test your message to be sure that your prospects understand your promise as such. If you wish to limit your liability to less than the value involved, be sure to specify the recompense you will pay. That recompense should be significant enough to make up for your failure to deliver or it may have little effect. Check with a qualified legal authority on advertising to be sure that you risk no more legal liability than you are willing to accept.

Adding Value

The primary purpose of promising value is to entice prospects to become customers for a transaction, but when loyalty is your ultimate purpose, you should plan to use communications to add value to consumers as well as to yourself. Your communications should be designed, tested, and proved successful in enabling consumers to make their best decision under the circumstances.

This requires, first, that you know the best decision for your potentially loyal consumers. Then you must become and remain that best choice. Continuous *superiority* improvement must be the order of the day. Finally, you must give consumers the information that will result in their making their own best choice: the benefits you offer. Helping them to think in terms of the benefits they are truly after, and to compare the benefits available from competing choices, should enable them to identify you as the best option for them.

Because some delay typically occurs between consumers' choice and their actual use of a plan or provider, you may have additional opportunities to use communications as a device for *adding* value to the persons you successfully attract. Some delay between enrolling in a plan and its effective date is normal; some lag between making an appointment and being seen, or scheduling a procedure and having it done, is typical. Physicians can add value to new patients, for example, by sending them a video showing the possibilities in patient/physician interactions that can produce the most information and benefit from a visit for both parties.[7]

In another example, Humana added 15 customer service staff to initiate calls to new enrollees in its Medicare HMO; the new step welcomed consumers to the plan, answered any questions they had, and scheduled their first visit with their primary physician. This preliminary contact helped to reduce Humana's 90-day defection rate from 13 percent to 9 percent.[8]

Providers can add value by providing information to scheduled patients that will help them confirm their decision to see the provider or to go ahead with the procedure for which they are scheduled. Most consumers are likely to have some doubts and anxiety, and interim communications can help allay both. Such communications may be sent out to patients to reinforce their confidence through information about the provider or the procedure and the benefits available. Giving patients sources of information they may use themselves can also help, such as names of local or Internet support groups or chat rooms, or supplying new patients with the names of veteran patients who are willing to offer information and support.[9]

In addition to confirming the decisions of new patients or members, communications can help them gain the most benefit out of those decisions. Health plan representatives or member volunteers can advise new enrollees on ways to facilitate access to services, information, and benefit coverage—on avoiding the hassles and stress that new members might otherwise experience. Providers' staff or volunteers can make encounters easier and more rewarding by sharing tips from veteran patients on where to park, for example, or the easiest way to get to the site, or ways to get the most benefit from specific treatments.

Enabling consumers to gain the most beneficial information from you can include making call centers, information lines, and Internet Web sites available in the interim between the intent and the act of membership or patient encounter. The advantage of such consumer-directed communciation is the provision of precisely the information consumers are interested in receiving at precisely the time they want to get it—just-in-time communications.[10]

Similar value-adding opportunities exist following patient encounters. One cancer specialist found that patients appreciate receiving a written summary of the diagnosis, treatment recommendations, and prognosis, all of which are being sent to the referring physician anyway.[11] Providers who make the effort to call or write recent patients to check on how they are doing add the value of demonstrated caring (and may teach the provider something that will help in follow-up care). Given the effect of frequent contact in promoting loyalty, and the fact that feeling ignored and taken for granted is the paramount reason for losing customers,[12] the combination of pre-encounter and post-contact communication can triple the customer's good impression of the actual visit.

Giving consumers a single, relatively permanent person to contact with questions or concerns is another excellent way to use communications to add value between encounters.[13] This can personalize a relationship with an otherwise impersonal and often intimidating organization such as a health plan or hospital. It can also give consumers a sense of a special personal relationship with a physician organization when they interact more with staff than with their physician.

Promises of benefits can actually add to customer perceptions of the benefits that they receive—and thus to the benefits themselves. The well-known placebo effect takes advantage of the mind-body connection to promote the beneficial consequences of treatment. In some cases, for instance, reliance on the placebo effect has been as effective as actual treatment protocols in delivering such subjective benefits as relief from pain and depression.[14] Further, the promise of particular benefits will prepare the way for consumer anticipation, thus heightening the probability that the promised benefits will be noticed when they occur (or missed when they do not).

Think of communications as a means of adding general value to the consumers whom you wish to remain loyal. Newsletters (easily customized to particular segments of members and patients based on their interests and health status) are a simple, inexpensive example.[15] The recognition of birthdays, holidays, and other special events in consumers' lives is a good way for plans and providers to express continuing commitment. And subsequent steps in the Loyalty Marketing Wheel will offer many more opportunities for building loyalty and reinforcing contacts.

When examined and used in context to promote and reinforce consumer loyalty, marketing communications takes on a wholly new and added significance. Although communicating begins with the challenge of enticing consumers to become patients or members, even this should be planned and executed with long-term loyalty in mind. In addition, you should communicate before, after, and between encounters to add value to and increase the contacts with the potentially loyal consumers you have in mind.

Connections

Promises can add to your impact in managing your organization as well as to the attraction and satisfaction you deliver to consumers. In areas where staff have been involved in discussing and agreeing on the benefits promised, for example, they are likely to feel a greater obligation to deliver those benefits. This has long been known as the "Avis effect," since Avis employees were actually found to "try harder" after an advertising campaign made that promise. Basically, this represents the Pygmalion effect, where people tend to live up to what others say about them.

Promise communications also prepare consumers for the next phase of loyalty marketing: the tracking and reminding steps. By giving consumers the confidence to expect particular benefits, promises can motivate consumers to monitor their own condition, looking for progress and benefits, for example, from the treatments and health enhancement programs that plans and providers have delivered to them. And once they are promised particular benefits, consumers are more likely to be prepared for a reminder about them—and are more willing to attribute the benefits to the reminder organization.

The effect of promises on tracking and reminding can be reversed to increase the impact of those promises. When you promote consumers' confidence in what they want and expect and in what you will deliver— the objective of promise communications—you may be able to add to consumer confidence by describing the ways in which you will track and remind them of the benefits delivered, in addition to your ways of delivering the benefits themselves. Filling people in on your complete plans for the use of loyalty marketing can promote their trust as well.[16]

The promise step in loyalty marketing connects the learning and management steps to the consumer, and enables you to perform the actual delivery of benefits that require the presence and cooperation of consumers. It then connects to the tracking and reminding steps, even as it veers backward to management by promoting both the delivery of added value and the enthusiasm of staff in delivering on the promise. The key to optimal use of this step is to focus on its full set of potential effects on other loyalty marketing steps and on the consumers who are its focus.

Figure 3-2 Communications Connections

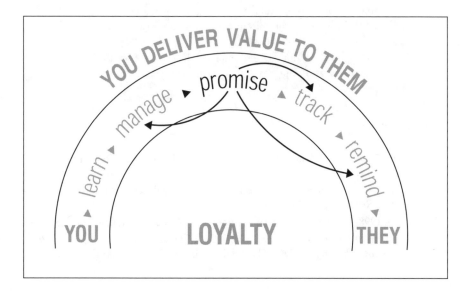

Action Recommendations

✓ Decide the benefits in your offer that you will explicitly promise versus the ones you'll leave as potential pleasant surprises to be tracked and used in reminders as they occur. Do not reserve any costs as surprises. _____

✓ Array the full set of benefits along a continuum of your confidence that they will be delivered. Select the benefits you will need to make your offer irresistible—the ones which you can afford to reserve as pleasant surprises when they occur. _____

✓ Separate the natural, current, and added-value elements in your offer for a clearly differentiated communications treatment. _____

✓ Distinguish between the "during" and the enduring benefits in your offer, and make this distinction clear in your communications. _____

✓ Cite past performance statistics, case histories, and testimonials as appropriate to promote confidence among prospects that they will gain the benefits in your offer. _____

✓ Describe the tracking and reminding system you will use, particularly when you lack much past history, to promote confidence among prospects. _____

✓ Carefully select the "promising" mode you will use to communicate your value offer, from description to suggestion to prediction to promise to guarantee, based on a combination of pretested impact and recognized risk. _____

✓ Develop your promises with the cooperation and enthusiasm of those who will have to keep the promises. _____

✓ Use communications in motivating staff to deliver on the promises you make. _____

✓ Use communications to prepare consumer perceptions of the value you've promised when they get it, and to confirm their choice before, during, and between your contacts with them. _____

✓ Use communications to add value to—and for—consumers, optimizing the likelihood that they will gain full value from their experiences with you, derive the full benefit and avoid inconvenience and costs wherever possible. _____

✓ Continuously monitor and strive to improve the effectiveness and efficiency of your communications, just as you do with your delivery of value. _____

References

1. Retsky, M. L. 1998. "Misleading Ads Could Be as Litigious as Outright Lies." *Marketing News* 32, no. 16 (3 August): 5–6.

2. Cohen, R. 1998. "Report Card Makes Its Mark at Long Beach Memorial." *Healthcare Marketing Report* 16, no. 2 (February): 1–3.

3. Baker, S. 1998. *Managing Patient Expectations*, pp. 37, 160. San Francisco: Jossey-Bass.

4. Health Care Advisory Board. 1990. *Successful Strategies to Increase Emergency Room Market Share.* Washington, DC: The Advisory Board Company, April.

5. "Currents: Managed Care." *Hospitals & Health Networks* (5 October 1995): 26.

6. Braus, P. 1997. *Marketing Health Care to Women.* Ithaca, NY: American Demographics.

7. Anderson, L., et al., 1987. "Effects of Modeling on Patient Communication Satisfaction." *Medical Care* 25, no. 11 (November): 1044–56.

8. "Currents: Managed Care: Spending on Savings." *Hospitals & Health Networks* (5 July 1997): 12.

9. Fell, D. 1998. "Customer-Centered Health Care." *Managed Care Quarterly* 6, no. 2 (spring): 9–20.

10. Peppers, D., and M. Rogers. 1994. "Welcome to the 1:1 Future." *Marketing Tools* 1, no. 1 (April/May): 4–7.

11. Damian, D., and M. Tattersall. 1991. "Letters to Patients: Improving Communications in Cancer Care." *The Lancet* 7, no. 338 (12 October): 923–25.

12. LeBoeuf, M. 1987. *How to Win Customers and Keep Them for Life.* New York: Berkeley Books.

13. Long, P. 1997. "Customer Loyalty, One Customer at a Time." *Marketing News* 31, no. 3 (3 February): 8.

14. "Placebo Effects Stunning." *Denver Post* (13 October 1998): 1A, 8A.

15. Padovani, G. 1998. "Mass Customized Communications." Presented at Alliance for Healthcare Strategy and Marketing Annual Advertising Conference, Chicago.

16. Karten, N. 1994. *Managing Expectations: Working with People Who Want More, Better, Faster, Sooner, Now!* New York: Dorset House.

TRACKING VALUE DELIVERED

Figure 4-1

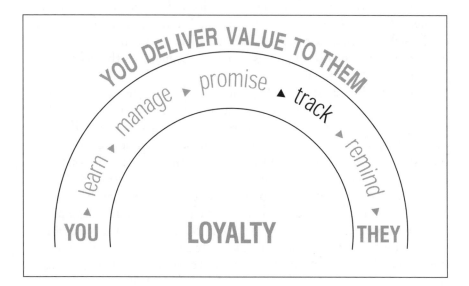

TRADITIONAL MARKETING, aimed simply at getting as many consumers as possible to buy as many of the marketing organization's products and services as possible, includes the three functions already discussed: learning about, managing, and promising value. The success of these functions has typically been gauged in terms of the number of sales, to the number of consumers and the amount of profit thereby gained. Given the maxim, "no margin, no mission," such success is by no means unimportant in healthcare. But it is not the end point for loyalty marketing.

When loyalty rather than sales is the focus of marketing, these three traditional functions require an additional two: tracking value delivered and reminding consumers of value delivered. Both focus on the value that has actually been delivered to consumers and on the extent to which consumers recognize that value and become loyal consumers and not merely satisfied customers. This chapter discusses identifying the value to track, the reasons why it should be tracked, and the best ways to do the tracking in the pursuit of loyalty.

Identifying the Value to Track

It is common practice to track the extent to which the promised structure and process elements have been delivered. Were patients seen within the promised 15-minute wait maximum, for example, or phones answered by member service staff within three rings? Did nurses smile and use patients' preferred names during interactions? Did member service personnel answer callers' questions without referring them to someone else? Such tracking is essential for management purposes, but it has little meaning in marketing unless the process includes the *delivery and perceptions* of "during" value.

In an age of evidence-based medicine and outcomes management, a natural and essential component of quality management is the tracking of outcomes. Certainly, outcomes are the *sources* for much of the value delivered by healthcare plans and providers. But clinical outcomes by themselves do not include the full extent of the impact that consumers enjoy (or suffer). Whether outcomes are measured in terms of absolute health status or its relative improvement or decline due to health services, they do not always affect patient satisfaction much; for example, in one study outcomes accounted for only 8 percent of the variation in satisfaction.[1] The effects of patients' impressions of "during" value and their subjective perceptions of benefits and costs seem to have far greater significance.

The primary focus of tracking for loyalty marketing is on value delivered. Given the definition of value adopted for this book (see page 3), the quantity and quality of life that consumers experience with value delivered is the consequence to be tracked. Tracking in this sense measures objective clinical outcomes such as recovery, cure, and longevity, which have clear value to consumers—and it measures subjective, personal values such as perceived health and functional status, happiness, and emotional, spiritual, and social well-being as well as physical health.[2] Given the potential of health plans and providers to have a dramatic and life-long impact on the quality and quantity of life for their consumer customers, it is astounding that so little has been done to track and remind people of the quality of life value they have gained through healthcare.

In addition to this enduring quality of life significance for consumers, providers and plans deliver a wide range of "during" benefits and costs. Although experiences during an encounter may be less important in the abstract, they can have a powerful effect on consumer loyalty at a time when the decision to remain a patient or member is made, and on the type and value of contributions that consumers make to their preferred plans and providers, that is, on their loyalty.

Does an encounter or contact with a plan or a provider reassure the consumer that this resource is acting in the consumer's best interests, rather than its own? According to a 1998 survey, 46 percent of consumers report a declining trust in health plans, 30 percent in hospitals, and 23 percent in physicians, so there appears to be plenty of reason to work on the "during" value that consumers perceive from their experiences with all three.[3] Do consumers, for example, accept—trust or understand—providers' bills, the reasons for provider choices of treatment, and the decisions of a plan in covering or not covering services?[4] Consumer impressions of particular experiences can determine their interpretations of long-term relationships with plans and providers and their decisions on continuing or dropping them.

Both in particular experiences and in lasting relationships, do consumers see the fulfillment of their needs, expectations, and wishes? Do they perceive, with either, any surprises—unexpected benefits that push them toward delight rather than mere satisfaction? Detecting positive surprises among consumers and tracing their causes can greatly enhance your loyalty promotion efforts. Consumers may well report benefits that surprise you as well as them, giving you wholly new ideas on benefits to promise as well as to track in the future.

Do consumers perceive any unexpected *unwelcome* costs that push them into the dissatisfied column? Early tracking can elicit complaints, suggestions for resolution, and redress of service failures or at least hints of their causes for future prevention. Discovering benefits promised but not delivered, or costs experienced but not anticipated, can yield the first indicators of challenges in creating and retaining consumer loyalty. It should also suggest the first order of business in recovering from service failures.

Identifying the benefits and costs to select for tracking requires careful thought. If you will spend time and resources to do the tracking yourself, you need to be sure it is worth your while. If you hope that some of your partners (employers, health plans, providers, other health-related organizations) will do some tracking, the benefits and costs must be both feasible and rewarding enough for them to track. If you expect consumers to track their own benefits, the ones you ask them to track must be significant enough to motivate them and appropriately identifiable to make it possible for them.

You should also select benefits and costs that are likely to be affected by your efforts to increase consumer loyalty. The satisfaction of scientific curiosity may justify some tracking, but because the purpose of the overall effort is to further consumer loyalty rather than to discover new knowledge, you should foresee some clear, practical advantages from the tracking effort and from the specific parameters to be tracked. This means that tracking should focus on benefits that are likely to be realized and costs that are likely to be reduced, so that findings will show that value has been delivered.

Awareness, Appreciation, and Attribution

Four dimensions of benefits need to be tracked:

- **Actualization** = the extent to which, in objective terms, they have actually and demonstrably been realized.
- **Awareness** = the extent to which consumers are conscious of benefits you have learned about, managed the delivery of, and promised to them, plus any that come as a surprise to you and the consumer.
- **Appreciation** = the extent to which consumers value the benefits versus the cost of the encounters, contacts, and relationship they have with you.
- **Attribution** = the extent to which they credit their encounters and relationship with you as factors responsible for the value they perceive they have gained, as opposed to other possible causes.[5]

Each of these dimensions of consumer-perceived value merits special attention, and all four together are needed for true success in your loyalty enhancement efforts. If benefits have not been delivered, their intended impact on loyalty is lost. If consumers are not aware of benefits, most of the loyalty value of delivering them is lost; if consumers do not particularly appreciate the benefits they are aware of, the effect of your campaign on loyalty will be small. And if consumers give you little or no credit for the benefits they are aware of and appreciate, you will gain little from achieving success with the first three dimensions. In this chapter and in chapter 5, approaches to both tracking and reminding consumers of value delivered will be recommended on the basis of their implications for all four dimensions.

Reasons for Tracking Value Delivered

The four basic justifications for tracking the value you deliver to the consumer are based on their importance to consumer loyalty and their actual effect on it. First is the fact that value delivery must be tracked in order to manage it well. Second is the usefulness of tracking value delivered in terms of marketing the value effectively. Third is the need to track value delivered in order to evaluate your own performance. Finally, the tracking of value delivery is essential to the next step in the loyalty marketing process: reminding consumers of the value they have gained.

Managing Value Delivery

Tracking value delivered is essential to the best job of delivery. If value is not measured to check on the extent to which it is being delivered, it can neither be managed nor improved. Without knowing the amount of value being delivered, there is no basis for improving either the effectiveness and efficiency of value delivery efforts or of initiating value improvement itself.[6]

Tracking value is by no means sufficient, although it is necessary for value delivery management. The right value must be tracked: the extent to which the value that was identified in the learning process, arranged for delivery via the management process, and promised in marketing communications has been demonstrably delivered and is perceived as value by consumers. Moreover, the linkage from benefits and costs back to the outcomes, processes, and structures that produced them must be ascertained for management to have the necessary information for proper action.[7]

Tracking can both enhance value efforts and enable management to further them. Tracking systems and results can be used as the basis for setting goals for staff and for monitoring and recognizing staff accomplishments in delivering benefits. It can be used as the basis for performance evaluation and reward systems. American Express, for example, rewards its merchant account representatives based on a measured amount of added profit value that has been delivered to their merchants.[8]

Marketing Value

Tracking value delivered also contributes to the most effective marketing of value. Tracking objective measures of value delivered can provide evidence—statistics, case examples, testimonials on value delivery success—for use in promising value to future prospects. Discovering what it is that consumers perceive as value delivered informs marketers of the benefits that are safe to promise and helps identify persons who are good prospects for testimonials, positive references, and enthusiastic word-of-mouth advertising (see chapter 7).

Moreover, tracking consumer perceptions of value delivered helps promote positive perceptions of that value and of the organization that delivered it.[9] Asking consumers for their impressions of encounters and relations with your organization will demonstrate your interest in their treatment by your staff and your commitment to good relations, often providing a "halo effect" on consumer attitudes toward your services. US West found that consumers who were asked by telephone about its services before they were surveyed by mail rated the organization 20 percent higher than those who were not phoned first.[10]

Evaluating Loyalty Marketing

Tracking the extent to which you can objectively demonstrate value delivered, and the extent to which consumers are aware of it, appreciate it, and attribute it as you wish, is essential to evaluating your overall loyalty marketing effort. You need to know not only the nature and extent of their value perceptions, but what kind of difference their value perceptions make when they are called on to show loyalty—both in attitudes and behavior. Xerox has documented, for example, that customers who rate themselves "highly satisfied" are six times as likely to buy again within 18 months as those only "satisfied." Obviously, it is critical to evaluate customers' feelings about the value they have gained and the organization responsible for delivering it.[11]

In other examples, Cleveland Clinic repeats Health Risk Assessments on its employer clients' personnel to determine the health risk benefits it has delivered to employees, while at the same time it tracks costs savings to the employers as well.[12] Promina tracks the number of patients seen within its promised 72-hour "reasonable standard" for appointments, and the number seen within ten minutes of their appointed time, to track improvements in waiting-time costs to its patients.[13] Aetna/US

Healthcare tracks the consumer health status outcomes of its health promotion efforts, as well as the impact of health promotion on clients' costs and the company's own profits.[14]

Evaluation, however, must go beyond tracking the improvement of particular performance dimensions through the delivery of value. It must include tracking the return on investment (ROI) of special efforts undertaken to improve the delivery of value, and even the ROI of tracking the value itself. How much better does your organization's performance become when you initiate a tracking mechanism for value delivery? It is not enough to *argue* that tracking is essential to management and valuable to marketing: evaluation should *prove* it.

Reminding the Consumer of Value Delivered

Although the next chapter is the one devoted to discussing the reasons for and ways to remind consumers of the value they have gained from doing business with you, it is well to remember that value tracking is essential to the reminding process. (Otherwise, what will you have to remind them of?) Moreover, two of the four tracking techniques that will be recommended shortly—namely, encouraging consumers to track their own value gained and surveying consumers about the value they perceive—serve to remind them via the tracking itself. Each time consumers assess their own benefits, through self-tracking, or respond positively to questions on perceived benefits, they are reminding themselves of value they have gained.

Time Lines in Tracking Value Delivered

For "during" value—the benefits and costs that exist only during and perhaps for a few hours or days after an encounter—the time to track perceived benefits, satisfaction, and other value indicators is during or soon after the encounter. You may also find it interesting to check some months later just to trace the decline with time of much benefit recollection and satisfaction.[15] Loyalty, measured as the intention to return or to recommend is particularly subject to decline when value has been delivered only during an encounter. In one example, only half of hospital patients indicated such intentions when questioned six months postdischarge.[16]

Durable value can be tracked later than the "during" variety and should be tracked more often. Your aim here is to avoid the risks that some consumer appreciation and attribution of durable value may fade with time, even when awareness is high. Consumers may simply forget about the time when they lacked function or gained its recovery, or they may lose the strength of connection to your organization when attributing the benefits they gained. Regular (but not nagging) reminders that generally ask former customers how they are getting along and specifically mention the problem they once had, can show your continuing concern for these consumers even as your reminders reinforce consumer recollection and connection.

Approaches to Tracking Value Delivered

Four approaches are basic to tracking the amount of value you are delivering to consumers and consumer levels of value awareness, appreciation, and attribution: (1) using your own records, (2) using partner/customers' records, (3) having consumers track their own value gains, and (4) surveying consumers on their perceptions of value gained. Each approach is worthwhile by itself, and each can substitute for or supplement one of the others.

Your Records

Your own records should be the best source of objective outcome data that reflect or suggest value delivered to consumers. Provider records can reflect improvements in objective measures of health status, in specific signs and symptoms, and in the use of healthcare attributable to timely and appropriate detection, diagnosis, and treatment. Health plan records can show reductions in health risks, claims, and out-of-pocket costs attributable to the plan's health promotion and demand management efforts.

The benefits you track yourself are those most suited for contingency reminding: benefits not promised, but potential pleasant surprises when detected. When other partners such as employers are involved, they may also cooperate in reminding consumers of pleasant surprises such as fewer missed days of work thanks to flu shots or an earlier return to work thanks to rehabilitation services.

The challenge for plans and providers is to translate objective clinical and claims information into value dimensions that clearly demonstrate their benefit to consumers. Some clinical measures, such as survival, restored function, and elimination of symptoms, are a fairly clear demonstration of benefit per se. Most others, however, will require some degree of translation. A dentist who proudly reports the reduction of a patient's gum pockets by an average of two millimeters is likely to be met with a blank stare—the patients want to know how much longer they can keep their own teeth!

Consumers may have a general appreciation of the importance and value of reducing their high blood pressure, cholesterol, LDL/HDL ratio, and many other clinical measures, but the perceived value of such achievements may be greatly enhanced by translating such clinical parameters into a mathematical reduction in risk of heart attack and stroke, or into improved prospects for longevity. Through such translations, the quantity or quality of life expectations for consumers are likely to be far more meaningful than the clinical measure itself.

Health plans must be especially careful in translating hard measures into consumer benefit. A report by the American Association of Health Plans reported that, on average, managed care organizations in 1996 had saved American employees $228 per person: $408 for married employees, and $191 for single employees. This may have been statistically true, but these figures were extrapolations of reductions in total health premiums from prior years and were not based on data that showed the proportion of these savings that had been passed on to employees by their employers. It was a statistical artifact rather than a true measure of consumer benefit.[4]

While reports of clinical measures may enhance patients' and members' awareness of clinical impact, they may produce little appreciation of the beneficial nature of the impact. With actualization, awareness, appreciation, and attribution all necessary for an optimal effect on loyalty, a maximum score of ten on actualization and awareness, and even with a ten on attribution, when coupled with a zero on appreciation yields a product of $10 \times 10 \times 0 \times 10 =$ zero impact on loyalty. Neither providers nor plans should assume that consumers fully appreciate the meaning and benefit of clinical parameters: they should ask consumers to describe the significance (if any) of the measures reported. This will enable the providers and plans to reinforce, correct, or initiate an appreciation of benefits that otherwise might not be perceived in their full significance.

When the persons closest to delivering the benefits are also tracking that delivery, the task can provide a continuing boost to their motivation. They may, of course, tend to bias their tracking in order to make themselves feel good (and to look good to any who might review their performance and reward them for delivering value). On the other hand, because objective measures of benefit should be used in this form of tracking, the risk should be manageable.

Your Partners' Records

Your partners and customers may be able to track some types of objective benefits better than you can. Some of the best indicators of success in a physician's case/disease management efforts may be reflected in the reduction of emergency room visits and hospitalizations that a partner hospital can track, or reductions in out-of-pocket expenditures a health plan partner can track. The success of a hospital's smoking cessation, or alcohol or drug abuse program may be tracked by physician monitoring of individual patients' blood, urine, or other health indicators. An employer may be able to gauge the success of a provider's or plan-sponsored flu immunization program by tracking absences compared to years when no immunizations were provided; the employers who do this will be tracking their own benefit as well.

Sports professionals and health club staff may be willing to track improvements in consumer performance—reflected in improved golf handicaps, tennis ratings, strength, flexibility, or aerobic fitness, for example—where the health plan or provider delivers such measures of benefit. Consumers may give some of the credit to the professionals or the health club, but the latter may well be partners in specific ventures with plans or providers to promote fitness in the first place. If sports/health club partners contribute to the measurement of benefits and the resulting loyalty of consumers, plans and providers can gauge the benefit of improved loyalty and lower-cost tracking against any reduction in attribution.

Consumer Self-Tracking

Self-tracking by consumers, via logs, diaries, and similar devices is likely to be the best (occasionally the only) practical method for tracking benefits for many provider and plan programs and services.[17] Weight management success can usually be monitored far more frequently by consumers than by providers or plans. The personal log or diary of the consumer who succeeds in smoking cessation most credibly can record the quitter's feelings from day to day as well as the length of time before he or she stops feeling the cravings and ill effects of nicotine withdrawal. Patients in depression treatment can record their level of optimism and energy each day.

The Cleveland Clinic, like many providers engaged in occupational health efforts, conducts annual health risk assessments on employees at client businesses in its corporate health program.[18] In addition to enabling the employer and the Clinic to track progress, the results of these repeated HRAs enable each employee to do so. It is likely that the specific parameters measured each year will require some translation so that consumers can fully appreciate the improvement in their health or the lack of progress.[19]

Encouraging consumers to track their own benefits, rather than relying on clinical measures and the interpretation of their meaning by others, has distinct advantages. Consumers can track subjective parameters more easily, since they are the subject. Moreover, there will be no questions regarding the credibility of reports, since consumers, themselves, are doing the tracking. They know best the value of their own good health.

A significant added advantage of self-tracking is the likelihood that it will reinforce compliance with medical advice and regimens. It is well known that getting consumers to track their own compliance helps in promoting that compliance, reminding them each time they record their performance of the next time to record it.[20] Imagine the added effect if they record not just their compliance, but the difference it has made to their quality of life whenever such an effect can be expected. Consumers may be willing to sign "contracts" agreeing to self-track their compliance if it includes tracking the benefits they gain thereby.

Recording their progress in weight loss, blood pressure, cholesterol, resting pulse, or other clinical measure changes, *particularly when they know and can simultaneously record the meaning of such measures in terms of quantity and quality of life,* can stimulate consumers to recognize the value of their compliance on a daily basis.

Such self-recording can greatly enhance a consumer's ongoing awareness of the benefits delivered. When consumers are well informed about the significance of the parameters they are recording, self-tracking promotes their appreciation as well. There is some risk, of course, that in recording their progress, consumers may downplay the contributions of plans and providers, giving themselves more credit for the benefits tracked than they deserve. On the other hand, a mixed attribution may be more realistic. It often happens that consumers' compliance with medication and lifestyle regimens becomes at least as important to the benefits they are tracking as are the advice and education of providers and plans. And consumers who consider themselves to be full partners in achieving health and quality of life benefits are more likely to be loyal than are those who feel wholly dependent and helpless.[21]

Perception Surveys

Some benefits can be tracked best via surveys of consumer perceptions—primarily psychosocial, spiritual, and emotional benefits rather than physical benefits—in instances where consumers' self-tracking of benefits is ineffective.[22] In cases of low or declining consumer motivation to self-record progress or compliance, when changes in beneficial measures occur only gradually, or when consumer self-tracking performance is poor, a survey can take the place of self-tracking. Even when self-tracking is successful, a survey may enable consumers to better fit their recorded day-to-day changes into the long-term picture.

In contrast to evaluation surveys, which focus on general consumer satisfaction and loyalty, benefit perception surveys address specific selected benefits, with the survey customized to the benefits the individual consumer is expected to perceive. Even though they are more expensive to design and administer than standard formats, benefit perception surveys are essential when consumers are expected to differ in the kinds of benefits they perceive. In addition to asking about the benefits for which you intend some perception by selected consumers (particularly those benefits promised and delivered), surveys should use open-ended questions to check on any other quality of life effects possibly noted by consumers. Empathic questioning and probing may discover unanticipated benefits and costs about which you should become aware.

As with postencounter follow-ups, benefit perceptions tracking should be used solely to track benefit perceptions. Although, for instance, it may be more efficient to use the survey phone calls to mention some service offered or a new plan option, this will tend to undermine the loyalty effect of the contact, making the tracking look not like an indication of personal interest, but an excuse, instead, to make a sales call.

Sometimes empathic observation can augment surveys to detect benefits of which consumers are only vaguely aware. Such observation was used, for example, to detect how proud parents became when their babies were able to use a pull-up diaper for the first time. None of the parents had mentioned such a feeling before; it became apparent only when they watched the babies' smiles and postures.[23] Surveys may have to guess about benefits such as the ability of a children's cough medicine to let parents (as well as their children) sleep through the night and wake up refreshed. The parents would then be asked if such benefits were part of the consumer experience.

Connections

The tracking effort should connect clearly and consciously to the other steps in the loyalty marketing process. Tracking itself is a learning step, and it should connect directly to the benefits found by the earlier learning step to be significant to consumers. The tracked experience should match the benefits to which management committed as well as the indirect benefits that were expected or hoped for. Most particularly, tracking should cover all of the benefits that were promised as well as those chosen as hoped-for surprises.

One marketing expert has described marketing as a series of closely connected challenges:

1. Ask customers what they expect (and want) from you.
2. Give them what they expect (and want).
3. (Tell them what they'll get so they will come for it).
4. Ask them if they got what they expected (wanted).[24]

Be sure you can connect the core challenges of each of your learning, managing, promising, and tracking efforts with each other, and eventually with the challenges you'll find in the forthcoming reminding and evaluating steps.

In addition, look for connections between the benefits you deliver and track—particularly those you verify to have been perceived as such by consumers—and consumers' subsequent attitudes and behavior in the return value chain. Learn the types of values and the levels of awareness, appreciation, and attribution that are first linked to identified levels of retention; then link them to the types and levels of contributions made by loyal consumers.[25]

By the same token, be sure to look for connections among the benefits you track—how the physical, social, emotional, and spiritual benefits connect to each other, for example. One study found that consumers still tend to define and judge their own health in physical terms. Their assessment of their physical health explained 55 percent of the variations in their overall health status rating, and the other dimensions of health, arguably as important, had no explanatory power at all.[22]

Figure 4-2 Tracking Connections

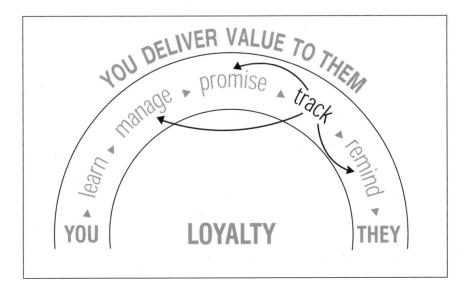

Action Recommendations

✓ Identify the specific measures you will use to track the benefits and costs you deliver to consumer customers, including your explicitly promised value and the benefits you've reserved as possible pleasant surprises. _____

✓ Ensure that the tracking system includes ways to identify unexpected benefits and costs (e.g., by including open-ended questions in surveys). _____

✓ Plan specific ways to use the tracking system in promoting consumer awareness of the value they have gained and, where possible, their appreciation and attribution of such value. _____

✓ Identify the value-tracking feedback you will gather for management's continuous quality improvement (CQI) efforts and determine ways to communicate such feedback to management. _____

✓ Identify the tracked value information you will use to validate or modify communications (and use as evidence for future communications), and the ways in which you will use such information in marketing communications. _____

✓ Track "during" value separately from enduring value delivered, and plan the timing of such tracking based on its delivery date and its time line of consumer perception. _____

✓ Combine your own records, data recorded by cooperating partners, consumer self-tracking, and consumer surveys to produce a complete picture of value delivered. _____

✓ Design your tracking system and prepare your tracked information to remind consumers of the value they have gained from your efforts. _____

References

1. Kane, R., et al. 1997. "The Relationship of Patient Satisfaction with Care and Clinical Outcomes." *Medical Care* 35, no. 7 (July): 714–30.

2. O'Donnell, M. 1998. "Observations from Our Founder." *Health Promotion: Global Perspectives* 1, no. 1 (March/April): 1.

3. Bagnell, A. 1998. "Becoming Customer-Driven: One Health System's Story." *Managed Care Quarterly* 6, no. 3 (summer): 28–39.

4. Brink, S. 1998. "HMOs Were the Right Rx." *US News & World Report* (9 March): 47–50.

5. MacStravic, S. 1998. "Don't Just Deliver Value, Demonstrate It!" *Health Care Strategic Management* 16, no. 8 (August): 1, 19–23.

6. Berwick, D., et al. 1990. *Curing Health Care.* San Francisco: Jossey-Bass.

7. Donabedian, A. 1966. "Evaluating the Quality of Medical Care." *Milbank Memorial Fund Quarterly* 44 (2): 166–203.

8. Whiteley, R., and D. Hassan. 1996. *Customer-Centered Growth,* pp. 12–13. Reading, MA: Addison-Wesley.

9. Bowen, J. 1987. "Using Surveys to Gain Insights into Service Value." In *Add Value to Your Service,* edited by C. Surprenant, pp. 45–48. Chicago: American Marketing Association.

10. "Customer Contact: Small Investment, Big Payoff." *The Marketing Report* (23 January 1995): 1–2.

11. "Customer Loyalty: A Critical Component of Long-Term Financial Strength." *Healthcare Strategy Alert* (January 1998): 1–5.

12. "Customer Loyalty Initiatives in Action." *Healthcare Strategy Alert* (January 1998): 6–8.

13. "Demonstrating the Value of Integration." *The Alliance Bulletin* (October/November 1995): 4–5, 7.

14. Wogensen, E. 1996. "Aetna Embraces Alliances to Handle Growing Complexity of Environment." *Strategic Health Care Marketing* 13, no. 6 (June): 3–4.

15. Bendall, D., and T. Powers. 1995. "Cultivating Loyal Patients." *Journal of Health Care Marketing* 15, no. 4 (winter): 50–53.

16. Fisk, T., C. Brown, K. Cannizzaro, and B. Naftal. 1990. "Creating Patient Satisfaction and Loyalty." *Journal of Health Care Marketing* 10, no. 2 (June): 5–15.

17. Cross, R., and J. Smith. 1995. *Customer Bonding: Five Steps to Lasting Customer Loyalty.* Lincolnwood, IL: NTC Business Books.

18. "The Cleveland Clinic Foundation: A Commitment to Strong Relationships." *Healthcare Strategy Alert* (January 1998): 7–8.

19. Prokesch, S. 1995. "Competing on Customer Service." *Harvard Business Review* 73, no. 6 (November/December): 100–12.

20. Baker, S. 1998. *Managing Patient Expectations,* p. 251. San Francisco: Jossey-Bass.

21. Morath, J. 1998. "Beyond Utilization Control: Managing Care with Customers." *Managed Care Quarterly* 6, no. 3 (summer): 40–52.

22. Ratner, P., J. Johnson, and B. Jeffery. 1998. "Examining Emotional, Physical, Social, and Spiritual Health as Determinants of Self-Rated Health Status." *American Journal of Health Promotion* 12, no. 4 (March/April): 275–82.

23. Leonard, D., and J. Rapport. 1998. "Seeing is Believing." *Marketing Tools* 5, no. 3 (April): 26–29.

24. Webster, F. 1994. *Market-Driven Management,* p. 88. New York: John Wiley & Sons.

25. Pottruck, D. 1987. "Building Company Loyalty and Retention Through Direct Marketing." *Journal of Services Marketing* 1, no. 2 (fall): 53–58.

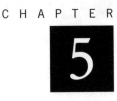
REMINDING CONSUMERS OF VALUE DELIVERED

Figure 5-1

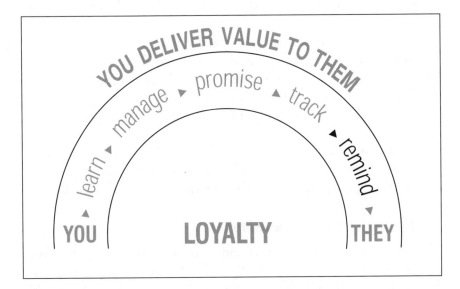

R EMINDING CONSUMERS of the benefits they have gained
from your services, a logical marketing communications task, is
commonly overlooked. To achieve the highest levels of consumer
awareness, appreciation, and attribution of the benefits gained from
particular encounters and from a loyal relationship, it is a good idea to

remind them of such benefits and not to rely on their own memory and perceptions. If much was invested in an advertising promise to attract new customers, it is worth some investment, certainly, to retain current customers by reminding them of past benefits.

Since tracking value delivered is essential to ensure that a promised benefit is delivered, it seems odd that so little use is made of the information gained through tracking. The potential payoff derived from reminding consumers of benefits gained lies in the loyalty effect that heightened awareness, appreciation, and attribution of benefit can have. It is impossible to pinpoint the investment justified in reminding consumers of past benefits compared to promising future benefits—only experience will tell its effects on consumer loyalty and the value of those effects to the organization. But it can be argued that some investment at least should be considered and tested to reveal the payoffs.

Reasons to Remind the Consumer

Numerous purposes, separate but related, can be furthered by reminding consumers of encounter and relationship benefits and costs. Eight are discussed in this chapter:

1. confirming the consumer's original decision;
2. promoting the consumer's awareness of benefits;
3. enhancing the consumer's overall perceptions of value;
4. inoculating consumers against rival efforts;
5. promoting the appreciation of benefits and attributing the benefits to you;
6. adding to the benefits perceived (placebo effect);
7. promoting confident expectations of future benefits; and
8. enhancing the pride and satisfaction of internal stakeholders.

Confirming Consumer Decisions

The most immediate effect of reminding consumers of their gains from your organization is to convince them that they made the right choice. This is particularly valuable for new converts, who may have doubts about the promises you made to them.[1] Demonstrating the accuracy and reliability of your promises by reminding your consumer customers of the benefits they have gained from your efforts should overcome such doubts if the benefits delivered match the ones promised. When the benefits you remind them of include some pleasant surprises, the confirmation effect should be even greater.

Promoting Awareness of Particular Benefits

In many cases, consumers will barely perceive the benefits they gain or will remember them for only a short time. By reminding them of those benefits, you can awaken perceptions that would otherwise remain dormant. Plan members who have used no services may be reminded, for example, of the peace of mind they gain through assured coverage of emergencies. Patients who avoided the flu this winter because they were inoculated early on will often have to be reminded of the differences that the immunization made, since no event occurred to make them conscious of their symptom-free season.

Loyalty-building perks and rewards—perhaps total money savings due to discounts or total points toward prizes for improved health and lifestyles—can remind consumers of the extent of their gains. Even better, remind them of the *durable* benefits they have gained: increased optimism, energy, general well-being; restored function or an improved ability to cope with a chronic condition; improved confidence and effectiveness in their self-care and disease self-management; a reduction of the need for healthcare, with its attendant emotional and monetary costs; a reduction of pain and interference with normal activities; and retained independence, for example.

Enhancing Perceptions of Value

Just as the good that men do is often interred with their bones while the evil is remembered long after (to paraphrase Shakespeare's *Julius Caesar*), so is it more likely that consumers will remember the "during" costs, the unpleasant events of encounters, more vividly and longer than many of the benefits. Yet most costs imposed by encounters, with the exception of malpractice, are of the during variety. By reminding consumers of the benefits you've delivered, particularly the durable ones, you can help them perceive a more accurate balance of benefits and costs, and thereby provide a better perception of overall value to them.[2]

Although both benefits and costs of encounters may be remembered, those of relationships may not.[3] Ideally, you will have identified, managed to deliver, and promised relationship benefits as well as encounter benefits. But no natural event occurs to prompt a consumer's recollection of relationship benefits; you must supply the prompt.[4] You can do so both by reporting to consumers and by asking them about such benefits (more on this later).

You should not limit yourself to reminding them of benefits, of course. Acknowledge costs, too, to show your awareness of them and your sensitivity to the need to explain and, if possible, make improvements.

Cost reminders can include apologies for unexpected costs and notice of your efforts to prevent or reduce the avoidable ones in the future. Two-sided messages (both costs and benefits) are valuable loyalty builders because they are more likely to be perceived as credible and in effect to enhance your reputation for honesty.[5]

Inoculating Consumers Against the Competition

Although the reminder step in the loyalty marketing chain focuses primarily on making consumers aware of the benefits and overall value they have gained, it is also possible to inoculate consumers against the efforts of rivals to promote awareness of your shortcomings. Perhaps you are higher-priced than rivals, and therefore impose greater out-of-pocket costs to consumers for deductibles, copayments, or premium contributions. If so, you can remove much of the sting from these costs by reminding consumers of the costs and the benefits that (you are convinced) make up for them, making the overall value you deliver appear to be the best deal for consumers. When you acknowledge these costs, but in the context of overall value, the messages of your competition lose their impact.

In addition, by focusing on benefits (that outweight the costs), your reminders automatically lessen the effect of your rival's communcations that focus on structural features, process events, or the attributes of either. You will also help keep your own organization focused on benefits because your own staff will be involved in tracking and reminding consumers of benefits rather than features, events, or attributes. It is unlikely that you will be tempted to revert to the "default mode" of dealing in structure and process once you and your patients or members and your staff are focused on benefits.

Promoting Appreciation and Attribution

Even when consumers are *aware* of the benefits they have gained via encounters or relationships with your organization, they may not fully *appreciate* the value of those benefits. Consumers may be made aware that they did not get the flu, for example, but they may need a reminder that they avoided suffering and achieved added days of work and wages or saved vacation benefits. Parents may need to be reminded of their extra days of wages or family enjoyment because their children did not get the flu. A greater appreciation of money saved may be produced if consumers are reminded that they were able to enjoy something otherwise missed—a vacation made possible from savings due to smoking cessation, for example.

Just as full discussion of potential benefits helps strengthen promises of benefits, so does full discussion of the meaning of benefits delivered strengthen consumers' appreciation. A health plan's summary of the emergency room visits and hospitalizations avoided because of its disease management success can greatly enhance consumers' appreciation of benefits. Consumers may appreciate the benefits of triage services more if they are reminded of the travel time and expense they saved, the waits and hassles of urgent or emergency care avoided, because they obtained and followed a triage nurse's advice.

In many cases, specific clinical measures of outcomes may not be readily appreciated by consumers. Reductions in blood pressure, for example, may mean more if they are translated into a reduced risk of heart attack and stroke. A Stroke-Risk Worksheet has been published, for example, that enables consumers to calculate a reduction in their risk of stroke in line with a particular reduction in their blood pressure. A ten-point drop in blood pressure may translate into as little as a 2.5 percent or as much as a 10 percent cut in stroke risk, depending on the index blood pressure numbers.[6]

It is somewhat risky to include indirect benefits that consumers might not otherwise be aware of or consider relevant to the direct benefits delivered. You need to be conservative in citing indirect benefits: overclaiming benefits that consumers do not attribute to your interactions with them will be as damaging to your credibility as overpromising benefits in the first place. On the other hand, you may be able to enhance consumers' perceptions of benefits by including the entire household's benefits, when available on your database.

In addition to their further awareness and appreciation of direct and indirect benefits, consumers will, through your reminders, increase the extent to which they give your organization proper credit. Unreminded, consumers may not give appropriate *attribution* to your role in the encounters and relationships that delivered positive results. By reminding consumers of such benefits, you also remind them that you are rightly and meaningfully connected to the benefits.

Moreover, once you remind consumers of the full extent and importance of those benefits—and of your delivery of them—the consumers will be less susceptible to the promises of rivals who might be trying to pirate them away. You can remind your patients and members of the long-term and comprehensive benefits you have already delivered; all that rivals can do is make promises of possible future benefits. Rival offers by definition include risk, but your delivery of benefits has proved itself, thus enhancing consumer confidence in the advantages you continue to offer.

Adding to the Benefits Perceived—and Thus Delivered

Thanks to the placebo effect, calling consumers' attention to benefits can, like promises of benefits, actually add to the benefits consumers gain from encounters and relationships. It can also enable them to recognize ongoing activities that are beneficial to their quality of life—the extent to which their efforts at lifestyle changes, self-care, and disease self-management have paid off in terms of avoided illness, crises, or injury and in savings of time and out-of-pocket expenditures. This, in turn, can help motivate consumers to persevere in their own quality of life improvement efforts.

Promoting Expectations of Future Benefits

Reminding consumers of the benefits they have gained, and thereby reminding them of the congruence between promises and delivery, will enhance their confidence in the availability of similar benefits in the future and in the reliability of your future benefits promises. When you remind consumers of past instances of pleasant-surprise benefits gained, you are also heightening their anticipation of additional such experiences in the future. Although a rival may be able to promise them benefits, consumers *know that you deliver them* and are likely to see less risk in staying with you than in switching.

You must be careful, however, with expectations of future benefits. You can continually meet expectations if you use your communications to *guide* consumer expectations not simply to promote them. Monitor changes in the expectations of loyal customers to be sure your loyalists do not become overly enthusiastic and exaggerate their view of your capabilities. Because these expectations can arise from their own excellent experience of value gained, you may need to temper reminders of such benefits.[7]

Affecting Other Stakeholders

Although with the reminder step the main focus is on consumers, it would be wasting an opportunity not to include reminders to internal stakeholders as well. The staff and partners of the organization can feel proud of the benefits you have delivered to consumers. Most people who choose healthcare as a career do so in anticipation that they will make a positive difference to others; reminding them of the benefits you have delivered to thousands of patients or plan members can enhance staff morale by making it clear that you are fulfilling your mission, not merely enhancing your margin.

Reminders to the general public, policymakers, and regulators may also be a good idea. Typically, the community benefit reports of not-for-profit organizations describe only the effort expended and money invested for the general good. Imagine how much more impressive it will be if you can also describe precisely the ongoing history of benefits to the community. Reports of overall reductions in flu cases, premature babies, chronic disease emergencies, and similar community outcome measures provide good public relations. Reports of positive effects on worker absenteeism, productivity, morale, and so on—and on consumer perceptions of quality of life gains from health promotion and disease management—should be even more impressive.

The Types of Benefits for Consumer Reminders

Promised Benefits

The chief topic for reminders is the precise benefits as they were promised in communications: the explicit outcomes and value described in the initial messages used to attract consumers to your facility, practice, or plan. Each of these benefits should have been clearly and unequivocally promised so that they were included in the confident expectations that brought consumers to you. They should then have been explicitly tracked via one or more of the four described tracking methods so that you have something documented for the reminders. Even if the consumers did the tracking themselves, or were surveyed for their personal perceptions, your reminders can include summaries of the results and trends derived from these sources.

Pleasant Surprises

These can include all of the additional direct or indirect value dimensions that you have tracked on a contingency basis and have found to have a positive effect on the consumer, provided that you can make a case for taking the credit or for expecting appreciative consumers to attribute such benefits to you. In places where you find many surprise benefits, you may well reserve some for later reminders, rather than including all of them in the first reminder. This is a way to create both the impression and future expectations of ongoing benefits that will continually increase.

During Benefits

Both objective clinical results such as an immediate relief from pain or the restoration of function, and subjective results such as feeling reassured that one is welcome, respected, and important, for example, can be included in reminders of benefits gained "on the spot." In almost all cases, benefits during an encounter will have been tracked by asking consumers to voice their impressions during or soon after the encounter that provided the during benefits. This means, of course, that they already will have been reminded once. In addition, such benefits can easily be included in a quarterly, yearly, or even multiyear relationship anniversary summary of benefits delivered.

Durable Benefits

Wherever possible, include both the objective and subjective indicators of those benefits that endure, as derived from both encounters and relationships. Long-term maintenance of lower blood pressure, lower weight, and lower cholesterol levels, with their implications for health risk and longevity, are good examples. Restoration of function and avoided disease or injury can also certainly be included, as should general perceptions of energy, optimism, and well-being that have improved or lasted a long time. All can be valuable in both surveys of relationship benefits and summaries of relationship impacts.

The Timing of Consumer Reminders

The timing of benefit promise communications can be crucial. The ideal is to send your messages at precisely the time when prospects will welcome and use the information to make a purchase decision. The timing of benefit reminders can also be critical—and for the same reason. Overall reminders of benefits gained since the inception of a relationship with a provider or plan are best communicated at times when decisions about extending or terminating the relationship are to be made.

When dealing just with "during" benefits, however, timing may be geared more effectively to the duration of those benefits. For benefits that do not last beyond the particular encounter, any reminders should come during or within a week or two after the encounter; otherwise, consumers are likely to have forgotten about their experience and a reminder will have no effect. For benefits that last a while beyond the encounter, specific reminders of particular benefits of the encounter may more safely be used later on. A combination of encounter-specific during benefits and relationship-general durable benefits can be used to summarize total benefits.

Reminder Frequency

The frequency of reminders should be a function of their number, significance, and time of occurrence. For major, immediately discernible benefits such as restored function, reminders can begin as soon as the results are known and continue, perhaps annually, as long as the benefit endures. For progress that is both significant and rapid, weekly, monthly, or quarterly reminders may be used as long as the progress continues. Such reminders will serve to reinforce consumers' motivation to continue their own roles in achieving improvement, as well as to remind them of benefits gained thanks to the provider, the plan, or both. Individual benefit reminders should be timed to fit the pattern of their delivery.

Overall benefit reminders, those representing the fruits of lasting relationships rather than specific encounters are best timed on an annual report basis. These can summarize all benefits of the most recent year, plus overall progress or preserved benefits since the relationship began. Only patients and members who have gained significant benefits need be reminded of them—but this should include all patients and members you intend to keep.

The Manner of Reminding Consumers

The reminder effects of self-tracking and of perception surveys have already been cited. These effects can be supplemented by including summary reminders of the results of both types of measurement in overall reports of relationship-long benefits. Such summaries can include reminders of consumer-reported satisfaction as well as perceived benefits, particularly when satisfaction ratings are improving over time. For self-tracked benefits, this means a possible total of four reminders: each time the consumer records the tracked benefit, whenever the consumer reports to you the benefits self-tracked, when you include a question about such benefits in a perception survey, and when you cite overall progress on that benefit dimension in an overall report. For surveyed perceptions, the last two reminders apply.

When surveys are used for reminder effect, as opposed to their more common use in evaluating satisfaction, it is essential to survey *every* consumer. Although a statistically reliable and representative sample suffices for evaluation, only those consumers who are surveyed will feel the reminder effect of being asked about their awareness, appreciation, and attribution of benefits they have gained personally. If you intend to use a survey as a reminder to all of your consumer customers, you will have to survey all of them.

Whether you or a partner tracks them, objective benefit measures can be included in regular reports of particular benefits, where they occur rapidly or dramatically, and in reports of overall benefits. Ongoing feedback from consumers regarding particular reports that they find helpful and meaningful will enable you to make such reports continuously significant to consumers and to your loyalty marketing effort. Continuous adjustments in the content and format for such reports can help keep them fresh.

The biggest question regarding ways to remind consumers of benefits gained is whether to create reminders of benefits particular to individual households and individuals or to use population-wide reminders. It is common practice for hospitals, for example, to prepare community benefit reports outlining all they have done for their communities, as part of their public relations effort and to preserve any tax-exemption privileges. Such reports mainly list the amount of effort and the resources that the hospitals have devoted to community benefits, rather than the beneficial impact that their investment has had. They seem to be awakening gradually, however, to the advantages of reporting the health status improvements achieved as well as the resources expended.

Health plans are beginning to report on the benefits they have delivered to covered populations as they become more aware of the greater effect achieved by tracking and reporting outcomes than by adhering strictly to reports of structure and process compliance.[8] Tufts Health Plan, for example, gives its employer clients access to information both on the direct effects of its disease management activities on employee health and the benefits to employers of reduced employee absenteeism and lower healthcare costs.[9] Cleveland Clinic summarizes health risk assessment changes across its employer clients' populations to demonstrate the value of its corporate health program.[10]

It is likely that population-based summaries or reports of particular benefits do carry a more dramatic effect than the individual patient reports, because they include the benefits gained by as many as tens of thousands of consumers. As such, these reports are likely to be of great significance to employers and governments or civic groups concerned with the health of entire populations. On the other hand, typical consumers who already have a relationship with a plan or provider are likely to be more interested in the ways in which they or their families have benefited than in the health statistics for an entire population. Consumers told, for example, that a plan's or a provider's efforts enabled 10,000 local residents to avoid the flu are likely to be unimpressed if they, themselves, suffered from it that year. They may even see such a report as a clear indication of misplaced priorities, if they were not among those who were immunized, or of incompetence if they were immunized and still got sick. Your challenge must be to stay ahead of the consumer's query: **"What have you done for me lately?"**[11]

Thus, although publishing reports of overall benefits delivered for individuals or households will be substantially more expensive and complicated than population-based summaries, the reports will likely be much more powerful. It is entirely a judgment call whether the additional investment is worthwhile in reminding individual consumers or households and sufficient to produce a significant enough return on investment in terms of consumer satisfaction, loyalty, retention, and contribution to your organization's performance.

Aside from Cleveland Clinic's use of repeated health risk assessments as a device for reminding participating employees of the benefits of the clinic's wellness efforts for them individually, it appears that few examples of individual benefits reporting have been published. Cleveland Clinic itself has not yet reported on the effects of such a reminder on employee satisfaction, loyalty, retention, or contribution—either to the employer who sponsors the health effort or to Cleveland Clinic. On the other hand, one physician, after getting annual accounting summaries detailing the growth in his net worth over the years, reportedly decided to use the same approach with the health status of his patients.[12]

Reminders to individuals of their accumulated loyalty benefits is a routine component of many frequent buyer programs. Airlines send monthly reports on miles accumulated together with the trips that consumers can "buy" with those added miles. Retail merchandisers send customers reports of points gained through their purchases and of their nearness to qualifying for premiums or gift certificates, in a strategy to entice them into buying enough more merchandise to get their reward.[13]

Reminders of benefits to individuals and households need not be made on an outbound basis to be effective. Consumers may gain access to benefit data via the Internet, through use of a PIN number to ensure the confidentiality of data and to limit access. Such an approach can save the costs of outbound reminders as it ensures that interested consumers will obtain the information they want at the time of their greatest interest. Moreover, this approach enables the organization to track the number of

Web site visitors, and to check on what information each visitor down-loads, thereby adding to organizational learning about what information is important to which customers.[14]

An even less costly option is possible when the benefits gained and costs saved by consumers are uniform and based on the number of encounters. In such cases, you may try empowering consumers to make their own calculations of overall benefits, in effect, creating a self-evaluation. For example, the Department of Veterans Affairs is opening up local ambulatory care clinics to substitute for its hospitals as sources of care for veterans and to attract more veterans to the VA system. In many cases, each visit consumers make to a VA clinic instead of a hospital saves considerable time and travel costs and stress. VA clinics could exercise a mass media option (such as regional newsletters) to publish simple tables enabling veterans in different designated parts of each service area to calculate their total savings in travel time, expense, and stress by listing such savings per visit. The designated areas would be labeled based on increments of time/travel cost savings (e.g., 10 minutes and $2.00, 20 minutes and $4.00, up to 120 minutes and $24.00), and individual veterans could calculate their own annual savings based on their number of visits to the nearest VA clinic.

Although the costs of such an approach would be far less than individual tracking and reporting, there are risks as well. Many veterans might not bother to make the calculation; some might forget the total number of visits they made. A wise use of this option would include both a check against a no-reminder approach, to be sure the reminder makes a worthwhile difference, and a check against a personal reminder approach to see if the more personal and expensive approach delivers a better return on the investment.

As noted earlier, such an approach applies only to *objective* benefits that you would otherwise track and report from your own or your partners' records. For subjective benefits that can be self-tracked, the low-cost option is to rely on the self-tracking alone, not on a compilation and report of individuals' tracking results. For benefits subject to reminders via perception surveys, the survey of each individual consumer or household remains necessary to achieve the full reminder effect.

The sensible approach is to test individual, customized reminders on a sample of the population of interest to check the effect on satisfaction, loyalty, retention, and contribution levels. The combination of effects should be readily translatable into dollar value to providers and plans, and that dollar value can then be compared to the dollar costs of the individualized reminder system. Where actual dollar impact cannot be captured completely, the Delphi process can be used to arrive at a consensus estimate.[15] If no precise estimates can be made, consensus can be used to estimate whether the dollar value of measured effects is at least worth the investment.

Unless you try an individualized reminder system on a sample of your population of interest for at least some of the benefits you have delivered, you cannot evaluate the difference individual reminders make as compared to overall population-based reports. And worse, you may discover that difference only by watching its impact when your rivals employ such an approach. Far better to test the approach yourself and let your rivals learn from you, to their regret.

Connections

The reminding step, which reflects the results of the learning, managing, promising, and tracking steps, sets the stage for the evaluation step. If reminding makes a difference, it will be in the levels of satisfaction and loyalty found in the evaluation step—then in the levels and types of value return contributions made by loyal consumers. And the evaluation step should include identifying specifically the difference that the reminding step has made.

Figure 5-2 Reminding Connections

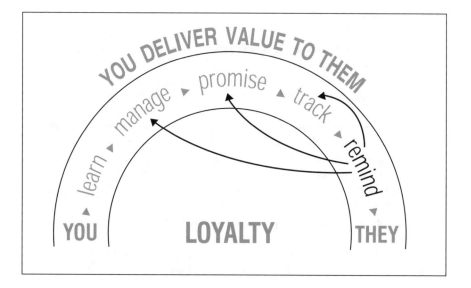

Action Recommendations

✓ Identify the specific objectives for your reminder effort to achieve, such as these results: confirmation of consumers' original decision; promotion of their awareness, appreciation, or attribution of benefits gained; an addition to their perceived benefits via the placebo effect; promotion of consumers' expectations of future benefits; and enhancement of internal stakeholder pride in the benefits delivered or in external stakeholders' attitudes toward the organization. _____

✓ Design the reminder process to achieve each objective selected, and prepare to evaluate the extent to which each is achieved (e.g., split tests to compare the reminder methods, control versus experimental group, to identify the value of the better reminding method to the organization). _____

✓ Select the consumers to focus on in your reminder efforts, that is, those who have demonstrably gained enough value to warrant reminding and from whom significantly greater contributions can be expected. _____

✓ Select the information content to use in reminder initiatives, from recorded data, self-tracked, and survey information. _____

✓ Select the media and timing of reminder communications for consumers and for internal and external stakeholders: customized or mass reporting, achievement-timed reporting, or annual summary reporting. _____

✓ Implement the reminder effort and prepare to evaluate its effects on consumers and on internal and external stakeholders; for instance, make sure you have "before" status measures of their perceptions and attitudes that you can use to gauge the effect of your reminder efforts.

References

1. Turk, M., and G. Kanely. 1995. "Brand Development: Implications for Success in Managed Care." *GrouProfile* 5 (2): 4, 8.

2. Peltier, J., T. Boyt, and J. Schibrowsky. 1998. "Relationship Building: Measuring Service Quality Across Health Care Encounters." *Marketing Health Services* 18, no. 3 (fall): 17–24.

3. Vavra, T. 1992. *After-Marketing: How to Keep Customers for Life Through Relationship Marketing.* Homewood, IL: Business One Irwin.

4. "Consumer Loyalty: A Critical Component of Long-Term Financial Strength." *Healthcare Strategy Alert* (January 1998): 1–5.

5. Baron, G. 1996. "The Four Stages of a Loyal Business Relationship." *Marketing News* 30, no. 19 (9 September): 7.

6. "Don't Have a Stroke." *Consumer Reports on Health* 10, no. 9 (September 1998): 1, 3–5.

7. Karten, N. 1994. *Managing Expectations: Working with People Who Want More, Better, Faster, Sooner, Now!* New York: Dorset House.

8. Graham, J. 1998. "Comparing Health Plans: The Search for Consensus." *Business & Health* 16, no. 9 (September): 58–64.

9. Goedert, J. 1998. "Tufts Puts Its Data to Good Use." *Health Data Management* 6, no. 7 (July): 44–46.

10. "The Cleveland Clinic Foundation: A Commitment to Strong Relationships." *Healthcare Strategy Alert* (January 1998): 7–8.

11. Levitt, T. 1983. "Relationship Management" In *The Marketing Imagination*, pp. 111–26. New York: Free Press.

12. Baker, S. 1998. *Managing Patient Expectations*, p. 251. San Francisco: Jossey-Bass.

13. "Bidding for Customers." *Cowles Report on Database Marketing* 7, no. 7 (July 1998): 1, 10–11.

14. Soljacich, R. 1998. "High-Tech, High-Touch." *Marketing Tools* 5, no. 3 (April): 30–33.

15. Delbecq, A., A. Van de Ven, and D. Gustafson. 1975. *Group Techniques for Program Planning*, pp. 83–107, 149–171. Glenview, IL: Scott, Foresman.

The Value Return Chain

Introduction to Part II

Part II completes the Loyalty Marketing Wheel discussion by presenting the return-value chain, covering the mining of consumer loyalty by eliciting consumer contributions to the organization. It begins with chapter 6, "Evaluating Consumer Loyalty," which addresses both the assessment of loyalty marketing success and the gathering of information to prepare for bringing about consumer contributions of value. Uses of the evaluation process and suggestions for conducting this evaluation are both discussed.

Chapter 7, "Promoting Return Value Contributions," covers ways to promote particular contributions of value by loyal consumers. First it presents eight categories of roles that may motivate loyal consumers and enable them to contribute, and twelve categories of performance that consumers may be able to improve for the organization. It then addresses eight basic categories of approaches to eliciting such contributions and suggests methods for selecting the approach best suited to the organization and its particular contribution challenges.

Chapter 8 discusses "Monitoring Return-Value Contributions." This is the return-value counterpart to tracking the value delivered to consumers, and focuses on assessing the value contributed by consumers. Described here are the advantages of such monitoring: to assess the effectiveness and efficiency of efforts to promote contributions and to prepare for recognition of contributions in the subsequent step. Specific suggestions of ways to monitor return-value contributions are then offered, together with examples of the likely sources and uses of the necessary information.

Chapter 9, "Recognizing Consumer Contributions," points out the reasons why you should recognize consumers' return-value contributions and ways to do it. Both consumer contributors and the organization's internal stakeholders are appropriate audiences for acknowledgment communications. Additional external audiences, including noncontributors and the general public, are recommended. Suggestions and examples of specific reporting and recognition approaches are offered in this chapter.

Chapter 10 addresses what may well be a controversial idea to many health organizations, namely, "Sharing the Value of Contributions" with contributors and the community. The essential logic behind this idea is the effect it can have on the sense of partnership and values alignment between an organization and its loyal consumers. Examples of the sharing strategies employed in other industries are presented in support of the idea together with examples of sharing programs in healthcare. This chapter concludes with suggestions for sharing value with both consumers and the community at large.

Finally, the epilogue offers a brief discussion of ways for you to complete the loyalty marketing loop and start another rotation of the wheel. Loyalty marketing is not a discrete process; it is an overlapping and ongoing process as it aims for continuous improvement in value delivered and in loyalty realized, and in the continuous growth of value returned by loyal consumers. Marketing for loyalty requires that the organization be consistent in loyalty to its consumers if it expects loyalty in return. It demands that both marketers and managers take on some challenging new tasks in order to realize success in mining the full potential of consumer loyalty.

EVALUATING CONSUMER LOYALTY

Figure 6-1

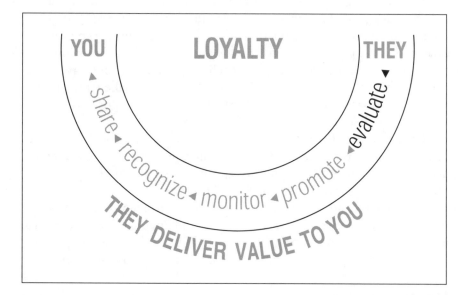

T HIS STEP, called "Evaluation," is actually a combined learning and tracking step, labeled differently to distinguish it from the first and fourth steps in the value delivery chain. In contrast to the previous "learning" step, it comes *after* the management and promising of value. In contrast to the official "tracking" step, it addresses the value *gained*

by the organization, instead of the value *delivered* to consumers. This chapter covers three issues: the reasons to evaluate, the signs of loyalty to evaluate, and ways to go about evaluating loyalty. The ultimate evaluation, that is, placing a value on the entire loyalty marketing process and specific initiatives, will have to wait until the value return chain and the entire loyalty marketing circle are complete.

Reasons for Evaluating Loyalty

Determining the state of your organization's relations with consumers is part of a "balanced scorecard" approach to performance assessment.[1] Gauging the consumer relations performance of your organization is as important as checking your financial performance. Possible performance measures include consumer satisfaction, turnover/retention, loyalty, complaints, and preferences—essentially anything that indicates your level of effectiveness in delivering value to consumers: in meeting and exceeding their expectations.[2]

One can list five management reasons for assessing the impact of loyalty marketing up to this point, and five marketing reasons for doing so. The management purposes served by this assessment are (1) to assess the return on investment gained from efforts up to now, (2) to examine each step in the process used to check if each adds value, (3) to consider the variety of approaches used in each step to see if any have been particularly successful, (4) to enable management to make strategic and tactical decisions at this point, and (5) to recognize and possibly reward those responsible for the success achieved so far.

The marketing reasons for assessing results at this point are (1) to determine the current state of loyalty of the consumers addressed by the marketing initiative; (2) to identify appropriate and superior prospects for value return contributions; (3) to identify the readiness of prospects to make general and specific contributions; (4) to identify any motivational, capability, or consciousness barriers and opportunities relevant to promoting value return contributions; and (5) to create among return value prospects a predisposition to make the desired contributions.

Management Purposes

1. Return on investment

The return on investment from loyalty marketing efforts up to this point will be the direct financial results achieved from gaining consumer business: bringing consumers in as patients and plan members. For management to have completed the five value delivery steps, consumers must have become customers, and presumably will have derived benefits subsequently tracked and used in a reminder process. In all but cases of charity and nonpayment of bills, this will have produced measurable financial returns: marginal revenue and margin contributions.

Clear and significant value in consumer satisfaction results may occur beyond the direct financial returns, particularly when such results are demanded by government regulators or business customers and are considered useful in marketing or public relations efforts. Checking on consumer satisfaction also prepares you to analyze the connections between satisfaction and loyalty. Satisfaction feedback can be helpful, too, in promoting internal morale and in guiding the management of service improvement.

In addition, if some degree of loyalty can be predicted, return on investment can include an estimate of future financial returns: premium payments times expected tenure as a plan member, monthly pmpm payments to providers under capitation systems times expected tenure as a patient, average fee-for-service revenue expectations per patient times expected tenure. Such expectations can be adjusted for the expected value of future money, and should use conservative estimates of tenure until long-term results of loyalty marketing efforts become known.

2. Value added at each step

Each of the five steps in the value delivery chain should add value to the loyalty marketing effort. The management, promising, tracking, and reminding steps that are based on the learning investment should be more successful than those lacking that initial step, and should be sufficiently *more* successful to cover the added costs of the learning effort. The promising step should pay off in greater volume and revenue than marketing would have without communications. Because of the evidence it makes available, the tracking step should show results in terms of improved management success in delivering the intended benefits as well as improved communications success. Tracking also provides the basis for the reminding step, and the reminding step should pay off in greater loyalty and tenure than would occur if no reminders were offered.

In practice, it is probably too unwieldy a task to conduct a thorough, scientific evaluation of each of these steps. The value of each cannot even be guessed until all of the steps have been completed, because the returns will not have occurred until then. And the only scientific means of assessing the impact of one element would be to conduct an experimental versus control trial of the overall process, with the experimental approach using the step in question and the control approach omitting it. This would make sense only if a particular step seemed either too expensive or ineffective, and management wanted to make sure it indeed was adding value.

3. Comparisons of approach effectiveness

When different approaches to specific steps have been used, it is important to determine the options that have been producing better results. For example, does an arms-length approach to learning produce better, equal, or worse results than a joint planning approach? Is one method for delivering a benefit more cost-effective or efficient than another? Does one means of communicating a promise of value—one based on testimonials, for example—work better than one based on statistics? Are data based on self-tracking as reliable as data from your own records and surveys, and are they less expensive? Do subjective surveys of perceived benefit achieve as much as surveys combined with objective data reports?

As with evaluations of each of the steps, checks on the approach to select for each step are best made on a control versus experimental approach or one that compares one "experiment" versus another, controlling to be sure that all other elements of the process are equivalent. This means that only one or two elements can be tested at a time in most cases, and that the ones most in doubt should be tested first. It also means that doubts about the steps themselves should normally be checked before checking on the optional approaches used in each step, although, to some extent, a test of a step automatically includes the particular approach(es) used to carry it out.

4. Midcourse management decisions

The point of evaluation (aside from published articles by the evaluators) is to enable management (1) to make midcourse corrections in the loyalty marketing process; and (2) to decide whether to continue, terminate, or significantly modify its targets, objectives, or investments. This purpose has significant implications for evaluation timing as well as content, and therefore for the methodology employed. Given the importance of management support in loyalty marketing and the shorter time frame most managers have to deal with, evaluation should ensure that management gets timely and relevent information to ensure that loyalty marketing initiatives do not die from neglect.

5. Staff acknowledgment

Finally, the identification of results and return at this point should enable management to recognize and perhaps reward those staff members responsible for any success discovered. Although performance evaluation systems may well be based on value delivered, as with the American Express account executives mentioned in chapter 2, evaluation of the return on investment achieved thus far will enable management to justify the level of recognition and reward.

Just as tracking the delivery of value enables management to share information with staff on staff contributions to consumers' quality of life, so also should gauging and sharing the significance of those contributions to the organization prove to be a source of pride to staff. As staff members learn the degree to which their individual and collective actions contribute value to consumers and gains to the organization, they become better positioned to manage such contributions themselves, so that both they and the organization can enjoy the fruits of "open book" management.[3]

Marketing Purposes

1. Identifying current consumer loyalty status

A thorough assessment of the loyalty status of consumers is clearly essential in loyalty marketing. The reminding step as well as part of the tracking investment are intended to pay off in loyalty and its long-term advantages rather than in immediate financial returns. Loyalty, as stressed earlier, is entirely separate from satisfaction even though the links are strong. You will need to specify the measures of loyalty–and the number of them—to assess at this point. Initial measures, however, are likely to focus on attitudes and intentions, and not on behavior, given the time that may be needed to assess actual behavior.

2. Pointing out the best return contribution prospects

In addition to the importance of assessing consumer loyalty as an indicator of the ongoing success of loyalty marketing, the information gained by identifying the number and type of consumers—and the extent of their loyalty to the organization—will go a long way in aiding the value return process. Where particular contributions need be sought from only a few loyal consumers, for example, knowledge of the most loyal consumers and therefore those most likely to respond favorably to a particular appeal, will enhance the effectiveness and efficiency of such an appeal.

3. Assessing contributors' specific readiness

In addition to identifying the best prospects for particular appeals, an assessment of loyalty can include assessments of the general and specific stages of those prospects' readiness to answer those appeals.[4] General readiness can be based on the positions of consumers as they change, in stages, relative to the strength of their commitment to the idea of contributing to the organization: how grateful, supportive, and committed to the organization's success and survival they rate themselves. Particular readiness would assess the stage of their readiness to engage in a specific contributory role with a particular performance benefit in mind.

4. Identifying barriers and opportunities related to promoting contributions

In addition to pinpointing their stage of readiness, marketing assessments can include learning about prospects' specific motivation, capability, and consciousness barriers and opportunities for contributing. In my own loyalty research, I have found that consumers vary widely in their receptiveness to particular contribution roles. Although between 80 percent and 90 percent of loyal hospital patients have reported themselves to be willing to engage in providing feedback and information (an advisor role) and to recommend the hospital and refer their peers (an ambassador role), fewer than 25 percent felt comfortable about serving on governing boards or standing committees (a manager role).[5]

Consumers have cited both motivation and capability as barriers to a favorable response to appeals for contributions. Capability barriers may be cited more often because they offer a better excuse than admitting that one does not care enough, but lack of time and perceived lack of self-efficacy (for manager contributions especially) seem to be the most commonly cited barriers. One can surmise that greater motivation could overcome some barriers, so both motivation and capability may well be addressed (see chapter 7 on promotion of contributions).

Consciousness is almost always a factor affecting the potential for return value contributions by consumers. If they are truly unaware of the wide variety of ways in which they can contribute, or if they simply forget a particular possibility at the most propitious time, they will need something more than the fact that they are motivated and capable in terms of that particular contribution. One can conclude that if they were motivated enough, they would not forget. Assessing their consciousness of possible contributions and of the organization's wishes will help greatly in designing promotional efforts.

5. Creating a predisposition to contribute the desired return value

Because assessments of the readiness for contributions and the barriers to making them focus on consumers who are at least somewhat loyal to the organization, and with whom a relationship already exists, the learning approach used in an assessment can often be one closer to joint planning and problem solving than to arms-length research. Once consumers see themselves as active partners in addressing general or specific organizational problems or aspirations, the learning process may gain more than just information about what it will take to elicit contributions.

The joint approach to learning can become a form of virtual negotiation, for example, in which participating consumers specify and pre-commit to the event or program that will involve them actively in a particular contribution.[6] This will affect only participants in the process, of course, although their suggestions may well help in designing approaches to nonparticipants.

Where the contribution is significant enough, it may prove worthwhile to invite as many consumers to participate as are needed to contribute. One of my clients used focus groups, for example, not simply as a research technique but to secure the participants' pre-commitment to using the service offer designed with their help. Over 300 consumers participated in focus groups and over 90 percent of them became customers.

The Effectiveness Elements of Loyalty

Satisfaction

The first item to include in the evaluation of an organization's effects on loyalty is the satisfaction of consumers with particular encounters and with the state of their relationship with the provider or plan. Conventional satisfaction research techniques can be used in this process, although it is essential to measure consumers' ratings of their relationship in general, as well as their reactions to specific encounters. With loyalty as the key focus, a satisfaction scale with a clear extreme upper end is advisable, something like "delighted" or at least "completely satisfied." The lower end may distinguish between extremes such as "very dissatisfied" and "disgusted," although either answer will indicate just about zero loyalty potential.

Perceptions of Specific Benefits

In addition to evaluating overall satisfaction, an assessment of an organization's effect on consumers should include checks on their perceptions of specific benefits derived from the relationship. The tracking and reminding steps should have ensured that consumers perceive the specific promised benefits that were delivered and tracked, and about which they were reminded. However, an overall assessment provides a check on the general and lasting perceptions of value: benefits net of costs. An assessment of these net impressions may be made separately by asking consumers to identify the benefits they have gained from the relationship; or it may be approached by asking the consumers to self-rate their level of loyalty and then probing into their reasons for positioning themselves at that level; or it may involve some combination of the two approaches.

The Dollar Impact

The dollar impact of both the number of consumer encounters and the percentage of consumers retained can normally be calculated or estimated from financial records. The *change* in these two measures attributable to the loyalty marketing effort up to this point would be the most objective indicator of the value returned thus far. In addition to these direct effects, the bearing they have on job security for employees, happiness of shareholders, stock prices, and similar parameters can be included.

The Emotional Element

Measuring the extent to which you have positively affected consumers' emotions or "share of heart" is a key component of loyalty evaluation. Satisfaction may be any mix of rational and emotional dimensions as reported by consumers, so special efforts are needed to get at specific emotional commitment. Asking consumers to indicate the words they would use in describing your organization to others and in describing the feelings of others about your organization are applicable projection techniques here. Asking consumers to describe their feelings during a specific encounter can elicit emotional content as well.[7]

Trust

The level of trust that consumers have in your organization compared to rival organizations is another indicator of loyalty. Determining the extent of consumers' interest in maintaining a lasting relationship with you in contrast to preferring variety or making a new choice will help in selecting prospects for further loyalty efforts. Among those interested in developing a relationship with your organization, determining their expectations and wishes for such a relationship can be critical both in deciding whom to pursue and in planning how to go about it.

Do consumers perceive, for example, that you are acting consistently and reliably? Do they assume that you are acting in their interests and not only in your own? Are they confident that you will consistently make the right decisions and behave in a competent and professional manner in your dealings with them? Or do they perceive you as one who is primarily operating for your own convenience and in your own financial best interests? How do they expect you to behave in the future relative to these factors?[8]

In addition, ask consumers who sense that they already have a relationship with your organization to describe the value they see in maintaining that relationship. Consumers feel more confidence in providers and plans with which they are familiar, for example, and thus are more comfortable in dealing with them. They may perceive better continuity and coordination of care from providers who are familiar with them. Avoiding the need to repeat the same information to a new plan or provider may be perceived as an advantage in keeping the same one.

Respect

Assessing the level of respect for your organization can be as important as gauging trust.[9] How do consumers rate you on quality dimensions, on reputation and image in the community, both in absolute terms and compared to your rivals? To what extent do they admire you and feel proud of their loyal-customer association with you? Such feelings can be powerful predictors of the likelihood that consumers will recommend you to their peers and refer prospects to you.[10]

Altruistic Motivation

Your need to identify the altruistic values and motivations of consumers —their desires to make a positive difference or to help others through contributing to causes personally important to them or to the community or to mankind in general—is vital.[11] This can help you determine both their potential contributions and your organization's best appeals, such as asking them to volunteer in your efforts to improve the health of the community or to donate to particular prevention or research programs such as AIDS or cancer prevention or early detection (see the next chapter). It can also prepare you to share the value of their contributions with them in the best altruistic fashion (see chapter 10).

Willingness to Act on Your Behalf

It is important to assess consumers' attitudes toward contributing to your organization's general success and survival and toward your organization's particular roles and performance outcomes. One study, for example, found that 90 percent of consumers were willing to recommend or refer others to their preferred hospital but only 33 percent were willing to change plans in order to ensure access to their preferred hospital. Providing feedback was a contribution that 80 percent of consumers were comfortable about, but fewer than 20 percent felt the same way about serving on a board or committee.[12]

In addition to learning whether and to what extent consumers are willing to make particular contributions, it is also useful to identify their motivations. Are they grateful for benefits received and looking for ways to reciprocate—to discharge a felt obligation? Are they driven simply by the desire to make a positive difference? Do they anticipate gaining self-esteem or social approval—or new skills they can use in their career? Or are they looking for opportunities to socialize with like-thinking peers?[13]

Knowing the degree to which consumers are motivated to contribute at all, the contributions they prefer to make, and the motivation behind their willingness to make these preferred contributions will go a long way toward helping to promote specific contributions. It will help both in targeting the right individuals for contribution appeals and in designing the most effective and efficient appeals.

"Grade" on a Loyalty Scale

Measuring consumer loyalty per se along some loyalty scale is an obvious component of loyalty evaluation. Such scales may be based on any mix of self-reported perceptions, overall preferences, and intentions for future behavior. Such intentions may be surveyed in terms strictly limited to consumers' "customer" intentions, that is, to continue or repeat the use of a particular provider or to reenroll in a particular plan, or they may include any number of possible additional contribution roles. They may be gauged in simple yes-or-no terms or along a scale that reflects the strength of those intentions. But note that when such intentions are included among measures of satisfaction with past encounters, they reflect satisfaction more than loyalty.[14]

A consumer's intention to stay with one provider or plan may be gauged along a "perhaps," "probably," "definitely," and "absolutely" nominal scale, for example, or on a percent of probability scale from zero to 100 percent. The strength of intentions and loyalty, for example, may be gauged in terms of the amount (if any) of added out-of-pocket premium or fee payment costs that consumers report a willingness to incur in order to get *their choice* of the plan or provider.[15] A combined statement of satisfaction with their plan/provider and of self-assessed intention may prove to be a better gauge of loyalty than either measure by itself. Some consumers may be highly satisfied, for example, but have become interested in another choice for variety's sake, while others may be dissatisfied but with no intention to change because they don't perceive any better alternative.[16]

Specific perceptions may prove to be better predictors of loyalty than loyalty scales themselves. Do consumers conclude that they have gained significant benefit *and that they have been an active partner in achieving it,* for example? Do they feel that they have some control over their relationship with you? Do they sense that you personalize your contacts and services in contrast to treating them like everyone else? Are they committed to your survival and success, and do they perceive that they can contribute to these outcomes? Do they expect frequent future contact with you and significant benefit from that contact? Are they happy in their choice of you as their provider or plan, and are they confident that they know ways to get the most out of you?[17]

You may also approach loyalty from the other direction by asking consumers how likely they would be to switch under stated circumstances. Would they change plans or providers if they could save $10 or more per month by doing so, for example? Would they change if their employer or physician recommended such a change? Would they switch in order to get free access to specialists or for faster or more personalized services?[18] How much more would they pay out-of-pocket or in premiums to be able to continue their relationship with you? Not only can answers to such questions gauge loyalty and warn of potential defection; they can also suggest your important weaknesses in giving consumers what they want.

Loyalty questions should assess the level of emotional attachment, affection, and degree of trust that consumers have relative to your organization.[19] Self-reports of consumers' intended behaviors when they are confronted with choices of provider and plan can reflect loyalty: Do they intend to check with you first when looking for specific services? Do they consider you their best source of health information?[20] Do they choose you above all others whenever they have a choice? Are they confident that you value and appreciate them? How loyal to them do they perceive you to be? Can they cite examples of your past behavior and expectations of your future behavior that illustrate your level of loyalty to them?[21]

You may simply ask consumers to rate their own loyalty on some polar scale ranging from total loyalty to a rival through a series of lesser levels of preference to total loyalty to you. Unlike satisfaction scales, however, which have long histories of statistical validation, loyalty measures require lengthy patterns of future behavior for validation. Satisfaction is a specific reaction to a particular past experience, whereas loyalty is a general attitude toward future behavior; the two are far from the same and, of the two, loyalty is by far the more difficult to measure reliably.[22]

Methods and Measures for Evaluating Loyalty

Because measures of loyalty include both objective and subjective parameters, a combination of objective and subjective measurement is required to gauge them appropriately. Objective parameters, such as the numbers of patients still active and plan members still enrolled, can be monitored in formal records. Actual behavior in terms of use of services or reenrollment in the plan are also found in records. The dollar value of retention can be assessed from financial records. Return on investment can be calculated by comparing the recorded value gained to the expenditures recorded for loyalty marketing. Clinical and other objective indicators of benefits delivered to consumers are obtainable from medical records and claims data.

Surveys are required, however, for the subjective measures of loyalty and of the impact of marketing efforts to this point. Simple measures of overall loyalty such as self-reported perceptions and preferences may be gathered through conventional survey sampling and survey techniques. However, as was true for the tracking of specific benefits delivered (chapter 4), both the kinds of survey methods employed and the numbers of consumers involved in a full loyalty evaluation will be quite different from what they are in conventional satisfaction surveys.

For control versus experimental comparisons, for example, you need reliable samples of consumers who received each of the "treatments" to be compared. This will at least double the overall sample size you need compared to producing an estimate of overall satisfaction or loyalty. To check the effect of including the reminder step on your consumer loyalty effort, a reliable sample of those who were reminded and those who were not will be necessary. If only a portion of consumers derived sufficient benefit to warrant reminding, separate comparisons will have to be made of those who gained minimal benefit versus those who gained significant benefit to see whether it was the amount of benefit or the fact of receiving reminders that made a difference to measured loyalty. This could mean double samples for reminding versus not reminding and double again for significant benefit versus not significant benefit.

Where internal split-tests of different approaches to a particular step are to be made, the sample size will at least double again. To check whether phone reminders work better or worse than written messages, you need reliable samples of persons who received both. To compare self-tracking or self-reminding to your own reporting efforts, samples of consumers who received each treatment will be needed, and you will want to find enough consumers who actually did the self-tracking/reminding. Otherwise you will not know whether any differences in results you find between the self-tracking/reminding group and those who received your reports are because consumers actually did not do the self-tracking/reminding as you expected, or to an effect that simply differs when consumers do it themselves.

In cases where different media and different message alternatives have been used in promise or in reminder communications, for example, reliable samples for each of the four mixes of treatments are needed, and the sample size increases fourfold. Where such different alternatives are used in both the promising and the reminding communications, sample sizes may have to be 16 times as large to detect the combined effects of all possible mixes of the different treatments.

Because different loyalty segments are likely to be of interest, additional sampling will be needed to obtain reliable information about each segment. Loyalty among women as compared to men; of healthy versus chronic patients or plan members; of different economic, social, ethnic, or age groups may have to be gauged separately, requiring adequate samples of each. Just establishing the proportions who are at different levels of loyalty and their differences from nonloyal consumers requires larger sampling.

To gauge overall consumer satisfaction as an organizational performance measure, for example, requires only a statistically reliable and representative sample of consumers, perhaps only 400 or so. But to gain all of the information desired from a loyalty evaluation will require surveying all consumers of interest. In order to identify precisely the best prospects for return value contributions, it would be essential to include every consumer in the survey who is likely to be loyal.

The sheer size of such a survey may make the loyalty evaluation process appear much too onerous and expensive to undertake, but you must compare the cost and effort expended to the value of the complete set of information you will have available to study. This full value can only be estimated at this point, since the actual value will not be established until the return value marketing chain has been completed. Where skepticism or scarcity of resources creates a barrier to investment in a complete loyalty evaluation, a deliberate subsampling approach may be used to pilot test the difference between having the full set of information on a sample of consumers in deriving return value and approaching another sample of the rest of the consumers without the information.

In addition to the effect of sample size on a complete loyalty evaluation, a significant impact also is likely in terms of the methodologies used in gauging subjective data and the expenditures required in doing so. Although standard survey techniques, including phone or mail surveys, focus groups, and depth interviews may be used for much of the general information, identification and commitment from the most likely return-value contributors is accomplished better through joint planning and problem solving.

This will mean using standard mass survey methods first, to identify the likely prospects, then inviting those prospects to participate in a joint effort to gauge their stage of readiness for making general or specific return contributions. Depth interviews, focus groups, virtual negotiation, and joint problem-solving approaches may all be applicable, singly or in combination, for particular segments of loyal consumers. Even though the costs of using such approaches for *all* selected prospects would be high, such costs would apply only to prospects whose potential return value contribution would make the investment worthwhile.

Satisfaction surveys focus on producing an objective numerical indicator of a single dimension, consumer satisfaction, or perhaps on loyalty indicators such as the intention to return or recommend. By contrast, loyalty evaluation is also aimed at discovering the precise number of identified consumers who are prospects for returning value to the organization. A sample survey may supply a basis for estimating number, but it will be inadequate for identifying and differentiating the best prospects. Moreover, in order to gauge the effect of the several steps in loyalty marketing, and of the different approaches to each, far larger samples would be needed than in simply measuring overall satisfaction.

The *process* of evaluating loyalty should be managed as one of the moments of truth that communicate to consumers as you gather information from them. You should plan and manage each survey to make the experience beneficial, cost-free, and easy for participants. Each should show that you already know the individual consumer; you should avoid asking them questions about how long they have been your customer or when they last contacted you. The answers, after all, are already in your records.

When you survey loyal consumers or prospects, consider that the questions you ask represent promises to respond to their answers. Plan to send a note thanking the respondents for their contribution of time and ideas, and reporting to them on your actions in response to any complaints or suggestions. Make as good an impression as you can in the survey process, and use survey materials and personnel who will convey the impression you want.[23]

These are suggestions only for differentiating the evaluation of loyalty from the evaluation of satisfaction or service quality. Given the many references on survey research and the impossibility of covering all of the techniques and tricks of the trade in one book, much less a chapter, my advice is that you consult one or more of the references listed at the end of this chapter or employ experts in survey research to conduct specific loyalty evaluations.

Some Caveats

Even though the focus of loyalty evaluation naturally is on the positive connections and contribution potential of consumers relative to your organization, the risk of negative impact is likely to be present—and worth gauging as well. Whenever significantly negative consumer attitudes are found, it is not wise to ignore them. Consumers have significant potential for doing harm as well as contributing return value, and when severely dissatisfied or disloyal consumers are found, they may be worth an investment to minimize the extent of harm they might do, even assuming that they cannot be brought back into the fold.

It has long been known that dissatisfied customers tend to tell significantly more people about their dissatisfaction than satisfied customers do about their satisfaction—an estimated two to five times more. In terms of getting an even balance of positive and negative comments, five times more means you need to ensure that more than 83 percent of your customers are satisfied simply to make up for the balance of slightly less than the 17 percent who are not!

Moreover, modern communications technology has multiplied—by orders of magnitude—the traditionally accepted potential for disgruntled consumers to tell 10 or 20 people about their negative experience. One particularly angry consumer can create a home page to share that anger with thousands, even millions of Internet browsers.[24] Moreover, other disgruntled consumers may hop on the bandwagon, adding their own vituperation to the first and promoting far more widely held negative perceptions than traditional word of mouth ever could.

Nowhere is there more risk of such an effect than in a plan's claims handling and a provider's billing and collections process. Perhaps because these functions seem to be managed from a predominantly financial paradigm, as compared to a marketing one, they seem to create a far more negative influence on consumer satisfaction and loyalty and very little positive impact. Billing errors, dunning letters that arrive well before insurance processes the claims, denied claims with weak or unclear justification—all not only annoy consumers, they impose anxiety, anger, frustration, and a lot of work on the consumers who are trying to get them resolved.

In addition to assessing the potential for positive contributions, you would be wise, as plans and providers, to assess the threat of consumer-caused harm in your overall approaches to risks in billing and collections and in your claims handling and loyalty evaluation processes. Rather than thinking in terms of the contributions consumers can make to the organization, think in terms of the kinds and amounts of difference consumers can make, both positive and negative.

Similarly, it can be just as dangerous to think about and approach consumers *only* as potential sources of contribution or harm, rather than to seek loyalty at least partly for its own sake. People do not usually wish to be seen and treated as a means to some end, but to be valued for their own sakes as individual human beings. Certainly it is true that most people are motivated by the opportunity to do good for others, including organizations they respect, but they are just as certainly capable of being annoyed and angered if they feel exploited and manipulated.[25] This reality is particularly important in selecting those consumers to approach for particular contributions and in determining the frequency with which to approach them. It will be discussed in more detail in the next chapter.

Connections

The evaluation step links back to each of the steps in the value delivery chain, as you check to determine the steps that have worked and how well, the impact each step has had, and ways to improve each step in the future. It also prepares the way for each of the rest of the steps in the value return chain, first as you learn the best methods to promote contributions of value. Evaluation sets the stage for monitoring the value contributed and gained by consumers. It should also teach you the most appropriate ways to recognize consumer contributors and the best ways to share gains with them and with the community.

Figure 6-2 Evaluation Connections

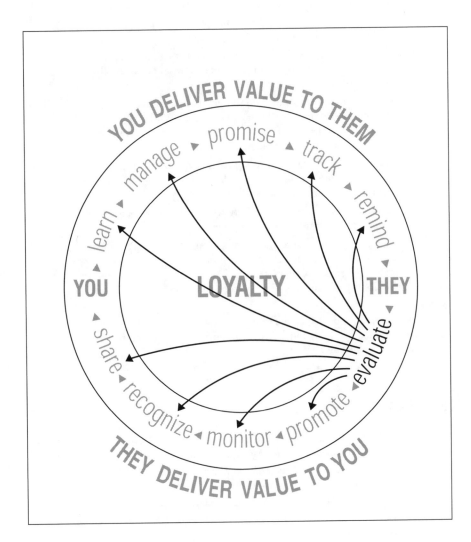

Action Recommendations

✓ Use the evaluation step to assess the impact of your value delivery efforts on both consumers and the organization. _____

✓ Begin with effects on consumers: their acquisition, satisfaction, retention, loyalty, and profitability of contributions to the organization. _____

✓ Extend the step to an examination of the organization's performance measures: volume, market share, growth, revenue, margin, public relations/image/reputation. _____

✓ Add the influence of value delivery on internal and external stakeholder perceptions and attitudes toward the organization, and estimate the worth of that influence. _____

✓ Use the evaluation step to check on the significance of each step in the value delivery process: the amount of value that each step adds to the overall results, for instance, experimental versus control group comparisons when one step is omitted or used for the first time. _____

✓ Use this step to check on different approaches to each of the other steps employed, for example, split-testing of different learning, delivery, promising, tracking, or reminding efforts to see if one works better than another. _____

✓ Use the evaluation results to contribute to overall management and to continuous improvement of the value delivery process. _____

✓ Use the evaluation process as the learning step in preparing for return value contributions from consumers: in identifying likely prospects with their stage of readiness, interests, barriers, potential, preferences for types of contributions, preferred methods for communicating appeals, and so forth. _____

✓ Select, collect, and analyze the information you need to achieve each purpose to be fulfilled by evaluation, and continuously assess and improve its level of success in achieving its purposes. _____

References

1. Sahney, V. 1998. "Balanced Scorecard as a Framework for Driving Performance in Managed Care Organizations." *Managed Care Quarterly* 6, no. 2 (spring): 1–8.

2. Karten, N. 1994. *Managing Expectations: Working with People Who Want More, Better, Faster, Sooner, Now!* New York: Dorset House.

3. Case, J. *Open-Book Management.* New York: Harper Business.

4. Prochaska, J., J. Norcross, and C. DiClemente. 1994. *Changing for Good.* New York: Avon Books.

5. MacStravic, S. 1994. "Hospital Patient Loyalty: Causes and Correlates." *Journal of Hospital Marketing* 8 (2).

6. ———. 1998. "Virtual Negotiation in Health Care Marketing." *Strategic Health Care Marketing* (May).

7. Day, R. 1989. "Share of Heart: What Is It and How Can It Be Measured?" *Journal of Consumer Marketing* 6, no. 1 (winter): 5–12.

8. Newcomer, J. 1997. "Measures of Trust in Health Care." *Health Affairs* 16, no 1 (January/February): 50–51.

9. Payne, A., M. Christopher, M. Clark, and H. Peck. 1995. *Relationship Marketing for Competitive Advantage.* Oxford: Butterworth-Heinemann.

10. Smoldt, R. 1998. "Turn Word of Mouth Into a Marketing Advantage." *Healthcare Forum Journal* 41, no. 5 (September/October): 47–49.

11. Izzo, J., and E. Klein. 1997. *Awakening Corporate Soul.* Fair Winds Press.

12. "What Makes a Person Loyal to a Hospital?" *Strategies* 3, no. 3 (undated newsletter published by First Marketing Company, Linn, OR).

13. Taylor, T. 1998. "Better Loyalty Measurement Leads to Business Solutions." *Marketing News* 32, no. 22 (26 October): 41.

14. Dawson, S. 1988. "Four Motivations for Charitable Giving." *Journal of Health Care Marketing* 8, no. 2 (June): 31–37.

15. Fornell, C. 1992. "A National Customer Satisfaction Barometer." *Journal of Marketing* 56, no. 1 (January): 6–21.

16. Gemme, E. 1997. "Retaining Customers in a Managed Care Market." *Marketing Health Services* 17, no. 3 (fall): 19–21.

17. Le Boeuf, M. 1987. *How to Win Customers and Keep Them for Life.* New York: Berkeley Books.

18. Sheth, J., and B. Mittal. 1997. "The Health of the Health Care Industry." *Marketing Health Services* 17, no. 4 (winter): 28–35.

19. Beckwith, H. 1997. *Selling the Invisible.* New York: Warner Books.

20. Levy, D., and M. Snyder. 1996. "In the Wired World, A Trove of Health Data." *USA Today* (6 March): 1D–2D.

21. Long, P. 1997. "Customer Loyalty, One Customer at a Time." *Marketing News* 31, no. 3 (3 February): 8.

22. Pruden, D., et al. 1996. "Customer Loyalty: The Competitive Edge Beyond Satisfaction." *Quirk's Marketing Research Review* 10, no. 4 (April): 24, 49–53.

23. Vavra, T. 1998. "Just Listen to Yourself: Poorly Done Satisfaction Survey Can Drive the Customers Away." *Marketing News* 32, no. 22 (26 October): 37, 43.

24. Stauss, B. 1997. "Global Word of Mouth: Service Bashing on the Internet Is a Thorny Issue." *Marketing Management* 6, no. 3 (fall): 28–32.

25. Reichheld, F. 1996, "Introduction" In *The Quest for Loyalty,* edited by F. Reichheld, xv–xxvi. Boston: Harvard Business School.

PROMOTING RETURN-VALUE CONTRIBUTIONS

Figure 7-1

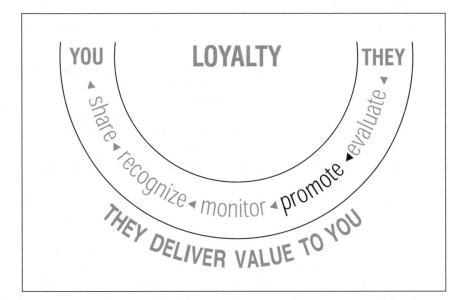

ARMED WITH information on identifying consumers, their motives for making particular kinds of return-value contributions, and the reasons behind these motivations, you are ready to promote specific contributions. Your first challenge is to match your evaluation-driven possibilities to the contributions you are most interested in receiving, that is, deciding on which identified contributions to appeal for. Next comes deciding the ways in which you will go after those contributions—putting together the sorts of appeals that will be most effective and efficient.

Identifying Contribution Possibilities

Although untold ways exist for consumers to contribute to your organization's performance success and survival, they can be examined in terms of a few contributory roles that consumers can play, and of the limited number of performance values likely to be of interest to your organization. Based on files of examples of the consumer roles that have made a difference historically (both positive and negative) relative to organizations, and a stock of readings as well as experiences in gauging organizational performance, I have identified eight role categories and 12 performance dimensions relevant to planning the promotion of return value.

Contribution Roles

The contributory roles of consumers now and in the past include the following:

- **Customers.** Consumers may buy or use your services or not, or may buy more frequently, a wider range of, or more profitable services. This is the traditional focus for relationship marketing.
- **Suppliers.** Consumers may serve, manage, or monitor their own health or act as caregivers for others in ways that improve the quality of outcomes or reduce the costs of care.
- **Volunteers.** Consumers may contribute their free labor to specific organizational activities and programs.
- **Donors.** Consumers may give money, blood, organs, perhaps goods of use to the organization (e.g., to be given to others in need or to be sold in fundraising efforts).
- **Advisors.** Consumers may offer up-front suggestions, participate in joint planning and problem solving, or contribute feedback on your own ideas and their experiences: they also perhaps provide "competitive intelligence" on the activities of your rivals.
- **Allies.** Consumers may take your side in political efforts to influence public policy or decisions made by other organizations.
- **Ambassadors.** Consumers may endorse your organization to others, referring or recommending your services to their peers, perhaps supplying testimonials or agreeing to serve as references on your behalf.

- **Managers.** Consumers may serve on your formal decision-making boards or committees.

This list can be telescoped into fewer categories by combining donor and volunteer, for example, because one involves donating things and the other donating labor. You can also expand it into more specific subcategories: customers by type of service used, suppliers by type of service supplied, donors by their donations, and so on. I have found that these categories are at least sufficient to stimulate a thorough consideration of possibilities without omitting significant options or carrying so many options that the analysis becomes paralyzed.

You should specifically address the fact that most of these roles have qualitative as well as quantitative ranges of possibilities. As a fee-for-service provider, you may wish for more customer activity among loyal consumers, while, as a provider or health plan at risk, you may prefer less activity and more self-care supplier contributions. When supplier roles are played well, they can contribute to higher quality and lower costs, and if played poorly, they can have the opposite effect. Consumers may engage in political activity contrary to your preferences or in negative rather than positive word-of-mouth: "bashing" your organization rather than endorsing it.

Any need to protect against and minimize negative "contributions" in addition to promoting positive ones is something your loyalty evaluation process should have helped you identify. General mass appeals to members, patients, or the public may reduce the tendencies of disgruntled consumers to create damage while they simultaneously increase the probability that loyal consumers will make positive contributions. In many cases, however, separately targeted attention will be required to accomplish these different purposes.[1]

Organizational Values

Although financial performance—and therefore financial contribution (reducing costs or increasing revenue)—is typically the contribution most frequently and fervently pursued, more and more organizations are recognizing the importance of using a "balanced scorecard."[2] Many marketing experts, for example, champion the idea of focusing on the delivery of value to customers and on gaining their loyalty, and weigh profitability as no more than the part of the scorecard used to reflect and reward the achievement of the first two performance dimensions.[3] In loyalty "mining," it is essential, first, to identify the performance dimensions or values that you are committed to improving and to maintain that balance.

After identifying the contributory roles on which to focus, it is helpful—perhaps essential—to bear in mind the particular performance dimensions or values that you intend to ask consumers to protect or enhance. This will help, first, in determining precisely the roles you wish for consumers and, second, in deciding exactly how they should perform those roles. Third, it may also help in motivating and guiding consumers as they carry out their roles, if they are committed to your success and survival, and to know the ends to which their efforts are to contribute.

The apparent organizational values that most organizations are pursuing fall into 12 categories:

- **Activity.** Volume of utilization, sales, visits, procedures, claims, and so on that represent both sources of revenue and demands on staff and systems;
- **Technical or clinical quality.** Objective, professionally defined and measured, adherence to own and others' standards;
- **Service quality or satisfaction.** Subjective judgments by customers that may be objectively measured for both internal management and external marketing purposes;
- **Productivity or efficiency.** Objective measures of the amount produced for the amount invested in labor, equipment, and supplies;
- **Operating costs.** Overall costs of conducting business, plus function or other specific costs, including medical loss ratio and administrative costs for health plans;
- **Revenues.** Actual collections, although "gross revenue" may also be tracked and compared to net collections;
- **Profit or operating margin.** The relationship between costs and revenues;
- **Mission achievements.** The measured good or the positive impact that the organization seeks and achieves in and for the community;
- **Relationships.** Status of the organzation's relations, reputation, or image with important "publics" or stakeholder groups, such as employees, shareholders, customers, suppliers, regulators, and the general public;
- **Market position.** Status of overall market size and of the organization's share in markets it serves;
- **Resources.** Status of key resources, from worth of assets to percentage of staff positions filled to age and obsolescence of facilities and equipment: reflections of the extent to which the organization has enough of the "right stuff"; and
- **Knowledge and information.** The extent to which the organization has the information systems and content as well as the organizational wisdom or learned skills needed to succeed and survive in rapidly changing markets.

Like the list of contributory roles, this list of organizational performance values or dimensions can be telescoped or expanded, and different terms can be used for many of the dimensions listed. These 12 dimensions should provide a sufficient basis for at least planning the kinds of contributions desired for most organizations, however, and they can be modified as needed by individual providers or plans. Recognizing that among the purposes of specifying these values is their possible use in motivating and guiding consumers toward particular contributions, it is important that they be both clearly and credibly presented.

Ways to Promote Contributions

Numerous reasons why people contribute value to others, whether individuals or organizations, have been suggested. Here is one list:

- **Reciprocity.** A sense of obligation or desire to repay for value received
- **Self-esteem/Image.** A wish to behave in a manner consistent with one's perceived true nature and values, or to become such a person through such behavior
- **Altruism.** A general wish to make a positive difference, to help others
- **Respect.** A motivation toward gaining social approval or acceptance, the respect of others
- **Personal development.** A wish to achieve something, perhaps to gain or employ existing skills and knowledge[4]

The evaluation step should have identified the mix of these motivations that applies to particular consumers, as a basis for your design of approaches to elicit contributions. Although the art and science of motivating people has a long history and wide-ranging theories of human behavior to work with, the actual methods used to get particular people to do particular things seem to be fairly limited. I have broken down all that I have used into eight categories:

1. **Asking, prompting, reminding, requesting, directing, insisting.** Any of a wide range of communications appeals that specify only what people are to do and when
2. **Persuading, selling, convincing.** Any of many communications appeals that are intended to motivate people to do something by explaining the reasons why they should
3. **Informing, educating, training.** Any communications appeals focused on giving people the knowledge, skills, or confidence (self-efficacy) they need to do something

4. **Rewarding, promising incentives up front, giving them after the fact.** Any means of making the desired behavior extrinsically more attractive and satisfying to consumers

5. **Marketing.** Any means of making the contribution intrinsically more rewarding, more convenient, or less costly for consumers

6. **Negotiating.** Discussions across the table of the desires of each side so that each will conclude that it will get what it wants

7. **Joint planning or problem solving.** Sitting on the "same side of the table" to plan and agree on goal-oriented activities for both parties

8. **Empowering.** Gaining agreement on or acceptance of the outcomes to be achieved through consumer contributions and leaving it up to the consumers to work out the actual achievement

These eight approaches are presented more or less in order of the time, effort, and risks related to their use. Each may be appropriate and more or less effective and efficient for particular consumers and particular contributions. Deciding the one to try first, and those to consider as fall-back or move-forward options, is often based on the importance and value assigned to the desired contribution, its desired time line, the number of consumers to take part, and the cost of each approach. Following is a brief discussion of the ranking of each of the eight approaches on these four selection criteria.

Asking

Often all that is needed is the simplest approach: to ask. When consumers are highly motivated, or if the contribution requires little investment on their part, a simple request that specifies what you would like them to do and when can suffice. Moreover, since asking is likely to take so little of your time and effort, you can afford to ask a large number of consumers in the hope that at least some will respond to the request: and if they total enough to yield the benefit you are after, then this may be the most efficient of the methods even with a low percentage of success.

Group Health of Puget Sound, in Seattle, Washington, for example, has used an "I'll Try Anything Once Club" of employees, physicians, and consumer members who agree only that they are willing to take calls and consider requests for particular contributions. The requests may be for stuffing envelopes, driving a homebound patient to a clinic, staffing a health fair, or any of a number of ad hoc purposes. Callers simply go down the list until they have the number of volunteers they need. The assumption is that the members of the club are motivated and able to respond to some appeals, depending on what the contributions involve and when the need arises, and that they will choose the ones to agree to.

For many contributions, a simple request may be all that is necessary, and it can make a vast difference in the numbers of consumers who make a particular contribution. A simple reminder to vote for or against a referendum may both increase the number of loyal consumers who vote on that referendum and the proportion who vote favorably; this is certainly preferable to a passive hope that they will do so. A simple request, for instance, enabled a lawyer to get ten times as many clients to make referrals as had been the case without the request.[5]

The key to successful asking often rests with the person making the request. Staff members of the organization who enjoy some kind of personal relationship with the consumer are likely to be more successful than strangers. Physicians may be particularly successful in situations where they have a close relationship with their patients. Opinion leaders, friends, family members, and coworkers may be successful with particular consumers, adding peer pressure to the normal influence of requests.

Persuading

In most cases, persuasion requires a good deal more effort per consumer. The assumption is that targeted consumers would be likely contributors if they knew the benefits that the act of contributing would have for them personally, or for their family, the community, some cause dear to them, or the organization itself. Persuading is somewhat arbitrarily defined and distinguished from the next approach, "informing," in an effort to differentiate the content as well as the purpose of the approach. Persuasion seeks to create or enhance consumers' *motivation* to respond, whereas asking relies on creating or enhancing their *consciousness* of the contribution to respond to, and informing aims to enhance their *capability* of responding.

Persuasion appeals may use any combination of benefit arguments or promises. The assumption here is that consumers made aware of these benefits will respond. These may be benefits they or their family will personally gain or benefits to their peers, the community, or mankind as a whole. In cases where consumers are committed to the success and survival of your organization, the persuasion appeal may involve benefits to the organization entirely. By first targeting those consumers who are fully capable of making specific contributions, a persuasion appeal aims at raising their level of motivation enough to elicit the desired response, while simultaneously making them conscious of that response.

Informing

Informing consumers is defined arbitrarily as using objective facts and information to create or enhance consumers' ability to respond to a contribution appeal. This may require some outbound education, telling them, for example, how to canvass a neighborhood to promote a new clinic or health fair, or supplying a self-care manual to enable them to care for more of their own symptoms. Some contributions may require hands-on training and practice for consumers to promote both their ability to perform and their confidence in that ability.

When the need is to promote consumer self-efficacy, that is, when they are already sufficiently motivated and conscious of the desired contribution, an informational approach often will suffice. Any combination of oral and written materials, of outbound and inbound communication, may work. A specific appeal may cite the contribution requested, then note that further information or specific training on how to make it is available on the organization's Web site, through a special phone line, or via scheduled sessions.

All of these first three approaches are based on communications alone. Each has a particular focus: on consciousness, motivation, or capability raising. Any mix of the three may be necessary and appropriate in practice. Depending on the loyal consumer's motivation, capability, and consciousness at the outset of the appeal, plus the complexity, frequency, and personal investment required in terms of the contribution requested, one or more of these communications-only approaches may suffice. And if this is the case, the desired contribution may well be realized at a minimal or at least reasonable cost and in a relatively short time compared to the more complicated approaches described in the next sections.

Rewarding

Rewards go beyond communications to change the nature of benefits that the requested contribution will return either to consumers personally or to altruistic causes. Promises of money, gifts, recognition, or anything that consumers value may be made up front to make the contribution more attractive, thus adding to consumer motivation. Even without such promises beforehand, some reward and recognition may be used to acknowledge a contribution made and to increase the likelihood of its repetition.

Although promising a reward may increase the proportion of consumers who will respond favorably to your appeal—and the delivery of a reward may increase the proportion of consumers who repeat the contribution—this approach has risks. It has been known for a long time that introducing extrinsic rewards for behaviors otherwise intrinsically rewarding tends to drive out intrinsic motivation.[6] The reward approach may provide a substantial success the first time or the first few times it is used in campaigns focusing on the same people, but its effects tend to diminish over time and the technique itself adds to the cost of the effort. Rewards are therefore best used for one-time appeals to minimize the risk that consumers will expect to be paid in some way for any contributions they make, although changing the particular reward for repeated contributions may slow the decline in impact.

A special type of reward is potentially usable by providers or plans, and it may achieve the added effect of a promised or delivered reward without the risk. Too few experiences have been reported with this approach to be sure of its effectiveness, but it appears to be a possibility. That approach is one based upon an altruistic reward. For example, American Express has used this approach by promising to donate sums to fight world hunger or on behalf of the Olympic Games for every card use. Cause-related marketing is frequently used in campaigns to boost sales.

If it works, in this narrow sense, for customer contributions used by purely commercial enterprises, it seems reasonable that the altruistic reward approach might work, perhaps even better, for organizations committed to community health and quality of life. (This assumes, of course, that your organization has, and is perceived as having, such a commitment.) The reward may be a promise to contribute some sum to a widely supported cause, or to invest in a community health endeavor favored by consumers. The fact that rewards go to the community rather than to the individual consumer may mitigate the tendency for consumers to feel that they are being "bribed" by personal incentives. It should be worth at least a try (see chapter 10, on sharing, for additional discussion).

Marketing

Like rewarding, marketing is aimed at making the act of contribution more attractive and satisfying, but it works on more than extrinsic dimensions. Through application of the marketing mix, it can include making the contribution more intrinsically beneficial, making it easier and more convenient, minimizing any costs involved to consumers, or any combination of the three. Although marketing may occasionally use extrinsic rewards (such as special discounts, prizes, etc.) in promotion efforts, its added potential lies in enhancing the intrinsic benefits of particular contributions.

Marketing may work on enhancing the intrinsic benefits that consumers gain in the *process* of making contributions: by including opportunities for socializing with their peers, gaining useful skills, and having fun, for example. The values that were discovered to be motivators in the learning step of the value delivery chain can be used as a foundation for designing and delivering as well as promising contribution experiences that will be perceived as irresistible by consumers.

In addition to enhancing the intrinsic benefits of particular contribution experiences, marketing can work on reducing any costs that might otherwise be involved. One hospital manager, for example, found that volunteers had to pay for their own uniforms and pay to have them cleaned, so the costs of volunteering could easily be reduced by buying and cleaning the uniforms for them. Even supplying pre-stamped envelopes in which to return survey questionnaires can make a difference in the numbers who respond. And with time costs often of greater concern than dollar costs, reducing the time it requires to make specific contributions is likely to increase consumers' probability of making them.

The convenience or ease of making contributions might also be enhanced. The hospital manager from the previous paragraph also found that volunteers who served before or after a full-time workday had to take their uniforms back and forth from home to the hospital. By designating an area and supplying hangers, the hospital was able to make it that much easier for volunteers. Offering multiple options for donors, from pledges and gifts to planned giving and estate planning, can make it possible for donors to find an option convenient for them; making blood donation possible at the worksite can greatly increase donations. Many ways such as these can provide donor opportunities.

In addition to marketing's improvements in the "product," "price," and "place" dimensions of contribution experiences, any asking, persuading, and informing communications, or a combination of them can be used to complete the marketing mix and "promote" contributions. In the true loyalty marketing tradition, such communications will emphasize the particular benefits versus costs that consumers will gain from the contributions they make, as well as the benefits that the organization will gain. You're well advised to use communications to add value wherever possible, especially through enabling consumers to gain the most value for themselves from the contribution experience.

The key to successful marketing is to keep both the benefit to consumers and consumer loyalty in mind as you work on getting prospects to make their contribution. Lying to them in an effort to make the contribution you want appear more attractive should be out of the question. So should threatening them or making them fear the costs of not contributing. Yet, unfortunately, dunning and the use of aggressive approaches to collect payments from patients, such as requiring cash deposits up front, are not only common but advocated.[7]

One of the physician groups I have worked with decided to begin charging interest (at the rate of 18 percent per year) on bills unpaid for 90 days. Since the group does not even send a bill to patients until their insurance has failed to pay for 90 days, this means that their first notice of the problem occurs when they get the bill with the threat of interest charges. The intention is to enlist patient help in lighting a fire under the insurance companies, but the effect is certainly negative to patient relations.

Easily the most egregious example of virtually extorting payments from consumers is that of the anesthesiologist reported to have required prepayment in cash of the $400 fee for epidural anesthesia by women in labor. Neither a check nor credit card payment was acceptable, so any woman who did not bring the cash was out of luck! Apparently the anesthesiologist felt that the Medicaid payment for the epidurals was too skimpy and wanted to make sure better payment was made, or else.[8]

By contrast are some of the more convenient, less painful ways of ensuring prompt payment. Many hospitals, for example, have worked to simplify and market prompt payment by accepting credit cards or arranging bank loans so that patients can take care of their hospital bills at the time of discharge. One system's Med Credit program used this point in promoting the benefit to patients of arranging payment promptly: "Helps you focus on your medical recovery and not worry about your financial recovery".[9] Whether patients actually found themselves feeling better off for having shifted their hospital obligation to a bank has not been reported, but the potential is there.

One truly enlightened marketing approach to handling patient financial obligations has been used by Franklin Memorial Hospital in Farmington, Maine. Patients who can't pay their bills are offered the option of working off their obligation as "volunteers," assisting with paperwork, data entry, working on the grounds, creating brochures— putting whatever skills they have to work for the hospital's benefit. Many patients prefer this arrangement to charity care and consider their unpaid efforts to be making a real contribution. They are ending up with a positive attitude toward the hospital, compared to the feelings of patients who have been aggressively pursued to pay their bills.[10]

Because the marketing approach focuses explicitly on delivering value to consumers in return for the value you hope they will contribute, it is the approach most suited to loyalty marketing. Should you choose to use this approach in pursuit of particular contributions, you need merely employ the value delivery chain with a focus on the particular contribution you are eliciting, just as you would with traditional customer contributions.

Negotiating

For high-value contributions that require a significant consumer investment and relatively few contributors, negotiations may be used. Face-to-face discussion or any number of fax, Internet, phone or e-mail techniques may be used in the actual negotiation process. The idea is that selected consumers sit, either literally or figuratively, on the other side of the table and thrash out an agreement involving the specific benefits they will receive in return for the specific contributions they will make. Although a legal contract could be the outcome of such negotiations, any agreement that results should be thought of as informal rather than enforceable, because the threat or use of force would undermine consumer loyalty.

The Farmington, Maine hospital described earlier, for example, refers to its offer of volunteer work to pay off bills as a "contract for care" program. No formal contract is drawn up, however, only the word of patients who participate. Farmington is a rural community where their word is still their bond. The very fact of an existing agreement, even an oral versus written one and even when it is unenforced, tends to promote the adherence of patients to the agreement.

Joint Planning or Problem Solving

This is an approach similar to negotiation, except that both parties literally or figuratively sit on the same side of the table and address the desired contribution as a common goal. This "virtual negotiation" approach includes all same-side, nonadversarial approaches where the particular consumer prospects for the contribution participate in designing the contribution experience.[11] In effect, the process examines as a joint problem the issue of what it will take to motivate and enable the participating consumers to make the contribution. Having taken part in its design, consumers are much more likely to take part in the experience.

This approach automatically delivers the benefit of shared power as it promotes the consumer contribution. As such, it adds both value to the consumers who participate and enhancement to the sense of partnership between you and those consumers. More than that, it gives you and the consumers an opportunity to learn more about each other, as you enhance the relationship through mutual disclosure.[12]

Empowering

Empowerment in this book also carries a narrow and arbitrary definition: to reach agreement with consumers on the outcomes, that is, on the particular performance enhancements to be achieved, and leaving entirely up to those individuals or groups the process decisions and activities that will achieve them. The agreement may be reached by simply asking for it—by persuading or informing consumers—in situations where the outcome is sufficiently motivating by itself. Incentives for achieving the outcomes may also be offered, with all of the caveats involved. Negotiations may be used to reach agreement on the outcomes, with the means left up to the consumers and not selected by the plan or provider.

The advantages of empowerment lie first in the possibility that you simply may not know the best way to achieve the desired outcome: consumers may have ideas you would never dream of. A second possibility is that multiple ways exist to achieve the desired outcome, and consumers who are offered choices can select one that they are comfortable with and need not accede to your particular approach. And third, enabling consumers to choose their own ways of contributing delivers the benefits of power, choice, and control, whereas the other approaches do not.

Selecting Your Approach to Promoting Return-Value Contributions

Both your organization and your consumers will be unique in each return-value contribution challenge, so selection of the best approach for prompting such contributions is a complex and difficult task. Your selection process should include at least an estimate of the costs and benefits of each approach: a reasoned estimate of the number of consumers who will contribute a specific amount of benefit if a given approach is used, and the amount of cost that will be incurred in time, effort, and finances to employ a particular approach. The approach with the greatest return on investment, or the one that comes closest to delivering the intended amount, will be your choice.

An alternative is to use an incremental approach, trying the least difficult and expensive first to check its level of success, and moving to the next in order until the desired results are achieved or the prospects of success are deemed too unlikely or expensive for you to continue. In addition to the level of success you reach with your chosen approach, this option has the advantage of enabling you to learn more about comparing the effectiveness of particular approaches with particular contributions and consumers.

When you initiate a loyalty mining strategy, it may be wisest to try the incremental approach first, since you may have too little experience, intuition, or information to estimate the costs versus benefits of particular options. As you learn more about the comparable advantages of selected approaches for particular situations, you may begin more confidently to select options based on credible and reliable estimates. In all cases, you should have reasonably accurate estimates of the value to your organization of achieving particular contributions, so that you can focus your learning on gaining a better understanding of the costs and the probability/rate of success that will result from particular approaches.

Connections

The promotion of consumer contributions of value rests on the knowledge you have gained through the evaluation step. The knowledge gained through evaluation then informs the monitoring step as you trace and examine the value contributed by consumers and the benefits delivered to them. Monitoring sets the stage for recognizing the contributions of loyal consumers. It may also presuppose value sharing if that step is used, either generally or specifically, in promoting contributions.

Figure 7-2   Promotion Connections

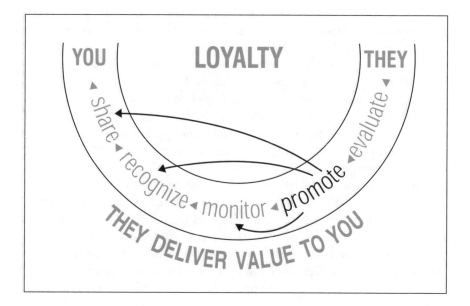

Action Recommendations

✓ Identify the types of contributions you are most interested in eliciting from loyal consumers, as customers, suppliers, volunteers, donors, advisors, allies, ambassadors, or managers. _____

✓ Identify the types of performance value contributions you want them to make to the organization, and all of the performance dimensions you wish to improve. _____

✓ Select the best prospects for the desired contributions based on the information you learned in the evaluation step. _____

✓ Analyze what you learned about their potential, stage of readiness, perceived barriers, and preferences in preparation for designing the approach you will make to them. _____

✓ Select the basis for the appeal you will make, the altruistic and personal values that you will use to elicit their contributions. _____

✓ Select your specific communications approach from among the available asking, educating, persuading, rewarding, marketing, negotiating, planning, and empowering options. _____

✓ Plan and implement the promotion effort to enable the effective and efficient implementation of the monitoring, acknowledging, sharing, and evaluating steps that will follow. _____

References

1. Hebert, R., and T. Reed. 1998. "Customer Relationship Management." *The Alliance Report* (May/June): 1–2, 10–12.

2. Sahney, V. 1998. "Balanced Scorecard as a Framework for Driving Performance in Managed Care Organizations." *Managed Care Quarterly* 6, no. 2 (spring): 1–8.

3. Dawson, S. 1988. "Four Motivations for Charitable Giving." *Journal of Health Care Marketing* 8, no. 2 (June): 31–37.

4. Reichheld, F. 1996. "Loyalty-Based Management." In *The Quest for Loyalty*, edited by F. Reichheld, ch. 1, pp. 3–16. Boston: Harvard Business School.

5. File, K., B. Judd, and R. Prince. 1992. "Interactive Marketing: The Influence of Participation on Positive Word of Mouth and Referrals." *Journal of Services Marketing* 6, no. 4 (fall): 5–14.

6. Amabile, T. 1998. "How to Kill Creativity." *Harvard Business Review* 76, no. 5 (September/October): 76–87.

7. "CEOs Say Patient Deposits Improve Cash Flow." *Hospitals* (20 February 1991): 48.

8. Bernstein, S. 1998. "Mom's Choice: Deliver Cash, or Bear Pain." *Denver Post* (15 June): 1A, 8A.

9. Nemes, J. 1991. "Hospitals Put Teeth Into Efforts to Collect Bad Debt." *Modern Healthcare* (17 June): 41–50.

10. Mehren, E. 1998. "Hospital Offers Low-Income Patients a Debt-Free Bill of Health." *Los Angeles Times* (8 June): A5.

11. MacStravic, S. 1998. "Virtual Negotiation in Health Care Marketing." *Strategic Health Care Marketing* 15, no. 5 (May): 3–5.

12. Darlega, V., et al. 1987. "Self Disclosure and Relationship Development." In *Interpersonal Process: New Directions in Communications Research,* edited by M. Rolloff and G. Miller. London: Sage.

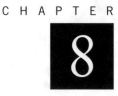

MONITORING RETURN-VALUE CONTRIBUTIONS

Figure 8-1

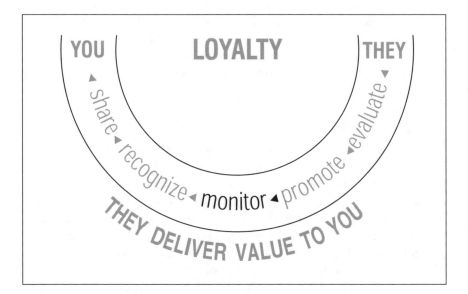

THE COUNTERPART to tracking value delivered to consumers is monitoring the value they contribute in return. This chapter describes the need for return-value monitoring, the contributions that call for it, and the ways in which monitoring is done for different types of contributions.

Reasons to Monitor Value Returns

Management Purposes

Value returns monitoring serves the strategic purpose of providing the information you need to decide whether the loyalty mining strategy is working. It also serves the same management purposes as the tracking of value delivered, in terms of helping to better manage the promotion of contributions, and it helps management become more efficient and effective by identifying what works well and what does not. Monitoring serves a purpose in internal communications as it enables you to report to internal decision makers the return on investment that is being gained from the overall value return effort and from particular contribution promotion initiatives. This should ensure that management is making informed and appropriate decisions regarding continuation of the effort. And it provides the basis for recognizing consumers for their contributions and for sharing the value returned with contributors.

A complete loyalty accounting system is needed, first, to track the total difference that loyalty achievement among consumers has made to the organization.[1,2] At a minimum, a modest increase in consumer retention should produce a significant, often dramatic improvement in profits and in overall financial performance.[3] Verifying this improvement and gauging the significance of the contributions loyal consumers have made to it is a minimum requirement for the return-value monitoring step.

Recognition Value

As with the tracking of benefits delivered, the monitoring of value returned also provides the basis for recognizing loyal consumers, reminding them of their importance to the organization. In instances where you have employed a marketing approach to promoting contributions—including some promise of benefits to consumers—monitoring should also gauge the extent to which such benefits were delivered to consumers and perceived as benefits by those who made contributions. For purposes of management, promising, and reminding,[4] you need to find out their degree of satisfaction with applicable socialization experiences, skills gained, and other intrinsic benefits promised and delivered.

The Return Contributions to Monitor

At a minimal level (the one most commonly practiced), checking on value returned means tracking the revenue and profit that consumers have produced for the organization simply by being its customers. How much have individual consumers bought or used, and how long has each been your loyal or at least consistent customer?[5] Quality monitoring systems are able to track both the gross revenue (charges) and the net revenue (collections) as well as the costs of serving individual consumers. Such information enables your organization to track the margin contributions of individual consumers as well as those of particular groups or segments.

In dealing with the full range of contribution roles and their effects on the relevant organizational performance dimensions, the challenge of monitoring becomes far more complex. At the same time, it is easier to track the benefits contributed by consumers, because you can use your own records for most of them rather than having to rely on a mix of consumer self-tracking, partners tracking, and consumer perception surveys. Monitoring any benefits promised to them in return for contributions to be sure the benefits were delivered and perceived involves the same tasks and approaches as the tracking step, step 4 of the value delivery chain.

Monitoring return-value contributions means measuring first the influence consumers have had on the affected performance dimensions. What difference have loyal consumers made to activity levels, revenue, quality, efficiency, costs, market share, relationships with other stakeholders, and any other dimensions?[6] Both the consequences for the measures that the contributions were supposed to affect and any implications or side effects for other dimensions need to be measured to the extent possible. If only the intended, presumably positive, effects are gauged and either positive or negative effects show up on other dimensions, you may mistakenly understate the costs and deem a contribution promotion effort a success; conversely, you may mistakenly (by understating the benefits) deem the campaign a failure.

In addition to measuring the effects of consumer contributions, it is essential to identify those consumers from whom they came. An initiative aimed at promoting word-of-mouth referrals by consumers and judged to have added 1,000 new patients or plan members, at a cost of $1,000, may be sufficient for you to judge the success of the initiative. It falls short, however, of enabling you to continue that success. Only by identifying precisely who among your loyal consumers made how many referrals— and perhaps by finding out how profitable or otherwise worthwhile those particular referrals were—can you learn which promotion approaches worked best and which had little impact.

Moreover, once you identify the consumers who made particular contributions and the worth of those contributions, you have both the information you need and the motivation to choose a way to recognize their contributions. You can remind them that you know how helpful they have been, thank them for their help, express your hopes for future assistance, and otherwise prompt them to repeat and continue with their contributions and their loyalty.[7]

Track back the contributions that particular consumers made to your original marketing effort that fostered their loyalty. What benefits delivered seemed to result in the best pattern of contributions returned—what reminding approach produced the highest value of return value contributions? The monitoring step should add to your store of information gleaned from the evaluation step as you continue to improve the effectiveness and efficiency of your loyalty marketing in general and your loyalty mining in particular.

Finally, only by knowing the specific consumers who contributed particular value returns can you decide whether, collectively or individually, you will share the gains you have enjoyed as a result of their efforts—and the best ways to share them. Just as traditional value delivery marketing is moving toward one:one customization for greater success in winning and keeping customers, so, too, does value return marketing need to use this same approach in mining the full value of such customers.[8] Maintaining a database on individual consumers, on value delivered to them and value returned by them, is essential to improve the success of individual initiatives and of loyalty marketing as a whole.

After identifying those consumers and the extent of value returned by way of their specific contributions, it is necessary to link the consumers and contributions to the kinds of appeals used to promote those contributions and to the evaluation-drawn information about those appeals. How well have specific gauges of loyalty predicted those who did versus those did not make any contributions—or particular contributions? How well did certain of the eight basic contribution promotion approaches work, given their costs?

While the ability to identify, evaluate, thank, and perhaps reward individual consumers for their contribution has the advantages cited, it also has at least two significant risks. The process of identifying the high-contribution individuals and recognizing their individual worth carries with it the risk that too much attention, recognition, and reward will be lavished on them to the exclusion of consumers who have yet to contribute to any extent. This may create a hierarchy in which some consumers get VIP treatment while others are ignored or given short shrift. Although this "tiered system" may help you maintain a loyal circle of high-value consumers, too many modest-value consumers not only might defect but might "defame" your organization as elitist and unfair, to your long-range detriment.

Moreover, with the increased recognition of the value-returning roles of consumers that go beyond their traditional customer role, the risk also increases that consumers and your relationships with them will be viewed merely as means to an end—their contribution value.[9] This can have a dangerous internal effect on your thinking and on your treatment of consumers, as you begin to emphasize their value as a means to your own good, rather than as a worthy end in itself. Not only can doing so threaten the entire loyalty marketing effort if such an attitude permeates your treatment of consumers, it can destroy the soul of your organization among its internal stakeholders and its reputation outside.[10]

To manage these risks, it is first essential to recognize the full *potential* value of loyal consumers, even if it takes more time to realize that value from some consumers than from others. Early high-value contributors may have helped your organization because of an early and significant gain that was a function of chance: perhaps they recovered dramatically from a heart attack as the result of the services your hospital's cardiac specialists provided; perhaps a life-threatening condition was detected early and cured because of your health plan's screening program. Many other potentially loyal and high-value consumers may be standing by until some similar event gains them a similar benefit. It would be foolish to drive them away through lavish attention to early contributors and inattention to everyone else.

The risk that relationships with consumers will be viewed and treated as means to a contribution value end is one of the most serious of relationship marketing myopias.[11] This is dramatically illustrated by the case of the physician who does everything right in promoting patient loyalty. Then, when a patient schedules tests at the hospital instead of in the physician's office (thus taking potential revenue somewhere else), the doctor becomes hostile, demonstrating that all of the friendliness and concern must have been a mere tactic to gain the most possible from the patient and not a true commitment to the relationship. The patient defects.[12]

Ways to Monitor Returned Value

Because the value of contributions to your organization's performance will be reflected in specific changes made or avoided in particular performance dimensions, you should find indications of returned value in your own performance records. By establishing baselines for performance parameters that you intend or expect to see improved, and remeasuring the parameters after consumer contributions have occurred, you should get a good idea of the effects that specific contributions have had. Simple before-after comparisons of the affected parameters together with estimates of the value of the differences should yield at least preliminary estimates of returned value.

A problem arises with this simple approach, however. Your performance parameters are likely to be affected by numerous factors: by other deliberate strategic and tactical actions, for example, as well as by competitor triumphs or blunders and other environmental factors. Assuming that the intended parameters have been affected in the right direction, how much of the improvement noted can you attribute to consumer contributions, and how much of the consumer contribution can you claim as the result of any recent loyalty marketing and contribution promotion investments?

Fortunately, tracking itself requires that you identify the total effects of contributions, the particular consumers who contributed and their contributions, and the specific promotion approach used to elicit those contributions. This combination provides the basis for attribution as well as evaluation of the effects. Tracking the effect of one referral on performance, for example, or of a representative sample of referrals where referred customers vary greatly in value to the organization, should provide a credible estimate of the value of each referral. Then, once the number of referrals is known and can be linked to specific contribution promotion efforts, the detected value difference can be directly and sequentially linked to the particular contributions, consumers, and promotion initiative that preceded that value difference.

A variety of scientific approaches, including the already described experimental versus control approach, can be used to make a rigorous case for attribution if this is necessary. In most organizations, however, a less rigorous case will be required, as long as *enough* value to cover their costs and represent a decent return on investment can be confidently attributed to the loyalty marketing and contribution efforts. In most cases I have worked on, the total value gain has been far greater than the investment made to achieve it. Because it makes practical sense not to claim dramatic ROI ratios that might not be repeated, it is often best to willingly share credit for performance improvements with other departments and initiatives.

In my experience, an ROI ratio of 1.5 or more is enough to satisfy most internal decision makers. Few other investments will return 50 percent interest a year. On the other hand, competing demands for budget allocations may suggest the need for a ratio of 2.0 or higher to gain additional funding for loyalty marketing given competing proposals and their ROI projections. Ideally, the total ROI *amount* rather than the ratio will tip the scales, but if you need to make a case for a high share of attribution in order to justify continuation, the full set of tracked information should help.

Otherwise, take the conservative route: both promise and claim relatively modest shares of demonstrated performance gains unless your need to aim higher is truly great. Promising more value than you need to gain funding and approval for particular initiatives merely puts you at risk of having to claim more credit for performance gains than you will be able to justify or of looking like a failure even if you can make a case for an admirable, but less dramatic return. Fighting for credit to gain a very high ROI not only will anger your colleagues but will also set the standard higher than you will like in the future.

If significant uncertainty or conflicting claims of attribution cloud the return-value tracking process, it may be useful either to bring in an outside expert or to employ a Delphi technique to reach consensus on the proper division of credit.[13] An expert may come up with any variety of splits, although if you can document a strong connection between performance improvement, demonstrated consumer contributions, and your promotion efforts, you should be in an enviable position when credit is allocated.

The Delphi technique engages interested parties in making a series of individual splits. Each participant's suggested split is melded with all others to yield an average split, and all persons whose splits are significantly divergent from the average are asked to explain the reasoning behind their opinion. Then all participants are asked to make another estimate of the proper split. If an outlier's explanation is persuasive enough, other participants may change their splits; if the outliers are unsure of their grounds, they may gravitate toward the mean. In any case, after a few rounds of this process, a group consensus usually is reached. If not, the last group average can be used. Not only is this Delphi method politically correct and fair, it also tends to be one of the more accurate means of estimating factors that cannot be reliably measured.[14]

Your aim in identifying these specific attribution links between performance gains, your overall loyalty marketing effort, and a particular contribution promotion initiative should be to gain credit for just enough of the value you have added to continue support of your efforts or any desired increase. Even if you can make a strong case for more than this, it will serve only to make you feel better in most situations and can threaten damage to your future efforts. This is not to say that you should aim merely to be "satisfactory" in what you accomplish, only in what you claim credit for.

Tracking Unrecorded Value

The comments in the previous section apply to the benefits you track using your own performance records. For at least some contributions, there will be no records you can rely on, and eliciting either self-reporting by consumers or surveys of their contributions will be necessary. Often, the tracking method is specific to the contribution made. Customer, donor, volunteer, manager, and advisor contributions will typically be reflected in your personal files: who bought, used, or donated what; who served for how long doing what; who complained, completed surveys, called, wrote, e-mailed, or faxed information.

However, for the categories of supplier, ambassador, and ally, at least, self-reporting may be the best or the only tracking method for some or all of the contributions involved. When a loyal consumer "supplies" caregiver services in a hospital's cooperative care unit, that is likely to be noted, for example, but it may not include all of the particular services rendered. The fact that daily costs of care and total costs per case are 30 percent lower in such units may be accepted as a reasonable measure of the value of consumer-supplied services in such cases.

But when consumers become suppliers of self-care or disease self-management services in their own homes, the extent and value of their individual contributions will not be recorded unless they record them or can recall them accurately in a survey. The overall value of self-care and self-management may be reflected in expense reductions among those who used a self-care or self-management phone line, received a manual, or completed training. The only way to know who actually used self-care or self-management and to estimate the difference it made in an individual case is to rely on self-tracking or reporting.

Self-care-motivated and capable consumers may be willing to track their own responses to symptoms when they arise or at least to estimate the number of times they used self-care when they would previously have gone to a provider. Self-managing consumers may record routine monitoring such as blood glucose levels for diabetes or peak flow meter readings for asthma. They may record in diaries or logs how often they experienced a particularly bad episode and what they did about it. This information can then be linked to utilization and claims records to see if these persons had fewer ER visits and hospitalizations, and lower total expenditures.

Absent the linking information about their use of self-care and self-management, even individual claims and utilization records showing less use of healthcare and fewer healthcare expenditures cannot be taken as a reflection of loyal consumer contributions. Reductions in use of a hospital's ER or inpatient care might merely reflect switching to another facility. Fewer claims might be accounted for by providers' own success in case management, rather than consumers' success in self-management. Self-tracking or self-reporting of supplier contributions may sometimes be necessary for value impact identification; they are almost certain to be needed for the attribution of such value.

Ally contributions—where consumers vote for or lobby others to influence decisions made by providers relative to plans, by plans relative to providers, or by governments, foundations, employers, and interest groups relative to plans or providers—are likely to be especially difficult to track and attribute. You may be satisfied if you identify increasing numbers of loyal consumers or higher levels of loyalty among them, then note that more favorable decisions are being made by outside organizations. But without connecting these two phenomena, you're not likely to know how much credit to give to your loyalty efforts or to specific get-out-the-vote efforts.

Some lobbying, by mail or by appearances at public hearings, can be tracked by consumers' forwarding of copies of correspondence, or through copies of the logs of hearings, including names of the speakers, for example. But identifying consumers who voted at all, or who voted on which side of which issues, is impossible to track objectively. Self-reporting is the only option for tracking most contributors as "political" allies. Like value delivered, ally contributions may be self-tracked and then reported, or reported in response to specific surveys.

For ambassador contributions, different tracking may be needed for different types of contributions. General enthusiastic remarks by your customers in conversations with others, or their recommendation of your organization when asked, may be trackable only through asking them to record and report when they do so or through surveying them to find out how often they recall doing so. Unless such surveys are frequent, you are likely to find that the responses either greatly understate such contributions (because of faulty memories) or overstate them (by consumers who want you to be happy with their answers and may feel that they should have recommended your organization when they didn't).

For actual referrals, you can ask new patients or plan members how they found out about your organization or happened to select it, then probing whenever the person mentions being referred by someone. Such probing should clearly indicate the reasons why you want to know, perhaps with something like "We certainly want to thank whoever sent you to us—could you tell me their names?" A combination of the referred consumer and the person who referred that new member or patient can then be reflected in your acknowledgment, thanks, or reward to the consumer ambassador, noting the name of the referred new customer and when he or she was seen or enrolled.

One physician combines referring, tracking, and rewarding by giving patients special business cards to hand out to their peers, with their own names as the referring patient signed on the bottom. All such cards that new patients bring with them are then put into an annual prize drawing for a free week in the doctor's time-share Palm Springs condominium. Only one lucky ambassador per drawing wins, although the others are rewarded with the opportunity. Other physicians have tracked referrers, then given a gift certificate for a free restaurant meal for two to all who refer five new patients.[15]

Monitoring Full Value

Upon identifying as well as you can the specific contributions of loyal consumers through any of their eight contribution roles, and the direct benefits to your organization attributable to the contributors, you should look to the indirect and extended value as well, just as you did in tracking value delivered. What good has increased volume, membership, revenue, and margin done for whom? What have self-care and self-management contributions and the resulting utilization and expenditure reductions done for whom? What good might they do in the future in addition to the indirect benefits already enjoyed? What is the expected effect of a contract signed or zoning approved that resulted from consumer political contributions, or of a new facility or program made possible through donations?

These indirect and future benefits may be important to a full appreciation of the value of particular contributions and of consumer loyalty in general. They may be needed to justify to internal decision makers the investments made or proposed for loyalty marketing. Or they may be useful to employ, as with the delivery of value to consumers, as pleasant surprises beyond the predicted and directly attributable benefits.

In most cases, whether these extended benefits are needed to support loyalty marketing investments or are helpful in gaining and maintaining internal support, they will be significant in the reminding step that follows, giving consumers a greater appreciation and pride in their contributions and giving internal stakeholders an appropriate appreciation for what consumers are doing to protect and promote the organization's success and survival (more in the next chapter, on recognizing value contributions).

Connections

The monitoring step feeds back to the evaluation step by validating your lessons learned about the best ways to elicit contributions from particular consumers. It also feeds back to the promotion step by assessing how well promotion efforts have succeeded for their costs and by testing which worked best when more than one approach was employed. Monitoring feeds forward to the recognition step by supplying the information, and it helps in the recognition process by reminding consumers, through asking, of some of the benefits they contributed and some of them they have gained. And finally, it sets the stage for value sharing by determining the value to be shared and its extent.

Figure 8-2 Monitoring Connections

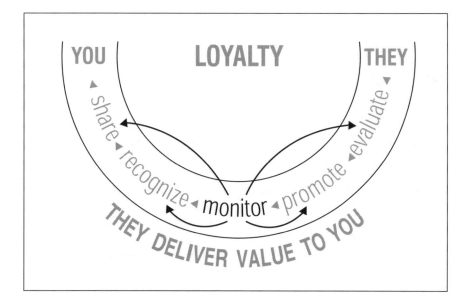

Action Recommendations

✓ Identify and evaluate the numbers of contributors and types of contributions loyal consumers have made to the performance value dimensions of the organization. _____

✓ Compare the value of contributions made to the costs of the contribution promotion effort and the cost of the overall value delivery effort, and calculate the return on investment. _____

✓ Assess which promotion efforts have been the most effective and efficient for identified consumers and identified contributions. _____

✓ Monitor the effect of contributions on the consumers who made them; ideally, this will show an increase in consumers' loyalty and motivation to make further contributions. _____

✓ Identify the consumers who made particular contributions of particular value in preparation for acknowledgment and possibly sharing in the value. _____

✓ Use your own records wherever they apply, but be sure to design other means of monitoring the contributions that will not show up in your records. _____

References

1. Merriman, C. 1998. "Marketing the Intangible." *The Healthcare Strategist* 2, no. 4 (April): 10–12.

2. Beckwith, H. 1997. *Selling the Invisible.* New York: Warner Books.

3. Reichheld, F. 1993. "Loyalty-Based Management." *Harvard Business Review* 71, no. 2 (March/April): 64–73.

4. Bell, C., and R. Zemke. 1992. *Managing Knock Your Socks Off Service*, ch. 15. New York: AMACOM.

5. Cross, R., and J. Smith. 1995. *Customer Bonding: 5 Steps to Lasting Customer Loyalty.* Lincolnwood, IL: NTC Business.

6. Duboff, R., and L. Sherer. 1997. "Customized Customer Loyalty." *Marketing Management* 6, no. 2 (summer): 20–27.

7. Bernstein, A., and D. Freiermuth. 1988. *The Health Professional's Marketing Handbook*, pp. 58–60. Chicago: Yearbook Medical.

8. Peppers, D., and M. Rogers. 1993. *The One to One Future: Building Relationships One Customer at a Time.* New York: Doubleday.

9. Bell, C. 1994. *Customers as Partners: Building Relationships That Last*, p. 132. San Francisco: Berrett-Koehler.

10. Chappell, T. 1993. *The Soul of a Business: Managing for Profit and the Common Good.* New York: Bantam Books.

11. MacStravic, S. 1998. "Marketing Myopia." *Healthcare Forum Journal* 41, no. 5 (September/October).

12. Stershic, S. 1996. "The Art of Relationship Marketing: Part 2." *Services Marketing Today* 12, no. 6 (December): 1, 5.

13. Karten, N. 1994. *Managing Expectations: Working with People Who Want More, Better, Faster, Sooner, Now!* p. 47. New York: Dorset House.

14. Delbecq, A., A. Van De Ven, and D. Gustafson. 1975. *Group Techniques for Program Planning,* pp. 83–107, 149–71. Glenview, IL: Scott, Foresman.

15. "Fun & Games Create Big Profits." *The Practice Builder* 11, no. 7 (July 1993): 1–2.

RECOGNIZING CONSUMER CONTRIBUTIONS

Figure 9-1

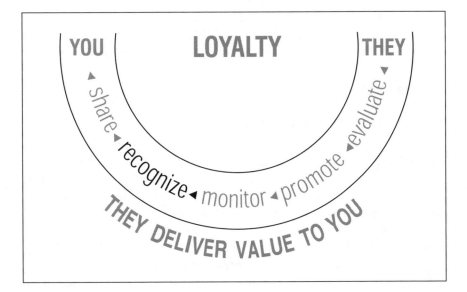

J UST AS the value delivery chain includes a step to remind consumers
of the value they have gained, so the value return chain includes the
step of recognizing, that is, reminding them of the value they have
contributed in return. And just as the reminding step includes reminding
other stakeholders in addition to consumer patients and members, so,

too, does the recognition of contributions include reminding consumers who are not contributors.

This chapter first describes the logical targets for reminding of such contributions, and the different purposes served by reminding different stakeholder groups. It discusses reasons why acknowledgment of the return value contributions made by loyal consumers represents an important step in the loyalty marketing process. It describes the different types of contributions to be acknowledged and the best ways to acknowledge such contributions to particular stakeholders.

Identifying and Recognizing Contributors

The principal, and obvious, group to receive your reminders of their contributions is the cadre of loyal consumers who have made them. Next come the latently loyal consumers; these are peope who so far have not made similar contributions but who might do so in the future. Third are the internal stakeholders, from staff employees to partner providers to boards and shareholders. Finally come the general population and external stakeholders whose attitudes and behavior toward you affect your success and survival. Since the issues behind recognizing consumer contributions tend to differ for each of these four groups, I will discuss each separately.

Contributors

Reasons to recognize contributors

The main purpose in acknowledging contributions is to make clear to the contributors that you recognize and appreciate those contributions.[1] Reminders to contributing consumers of your awareness of their help at least, but preferably also your appreciation and attribution of significant value to their efforts, shows that you are conscious of contributors' importance to you and that you want them to feel appreciated and valued.[2]

Such recognition will help to give loyal consumers a sense of sharing in your success through their contributions and of a partnership in your aspirations and achievements.[3] It provides a logical opportunity to thank them for their contributions and, by singling out each person, to promote the repetition and continuation of contributory behaviors.[4] One marketer found that customers who were simply thanked for their purchases increased their subsequent purchases by 70 percent, whereas customers who were thanked and told of special offers as well increased their purchases by only 30 percent, and customers who were not thanked did not increase their purchases at all.[5] This further illustrates the risks in loyalty marketing of treating customers as means versus ends and of causing consumers to perceive that they are being so treated.

Acknowledging consumer contributions should by itself increase consumer feelings of loyalty. This phenomenon has long been reflected in the increased probability that consumers who make one type of contribution will make other types as well.[6] This may be due to cognitive dissonance: since consumer behaviors demonstrate their loyalty to the organization, making further contributions would be consistent with that loyalty, while not making contributions or doing the organization harm would be dissonant. In any case, it is well known that people tend to make their attitudes and behavior consistent, so each affects the other.

For example, PacifiCare in Cypress, California has recruited members of its Medicare HMO, Secure Horizons, to become volunteers in its "ambassador program" since 1995. Two hundred ambassadors review and advise the HMO on member materials, make calls to new members, visit with them at enrollment and health fairs, participate in senior events, advise new members on how to obtain coverage and services, answer their questions, and help them learn the ropes as new members as they welcome them into the fold. They mainly use their own phones, preferring to make their contacts personal rather than business gestures.[7]

The use of these ambassadors has helped Secure Horizons expand the scope of its marketing communcations, and add to the value it offers new enrollees. According to PacifiCare staff, the program is so popular that it has a waiting list; it is featured in advertising as an added quality of life value element offered by the HMO: an opportunity for members to socialize with and make a difference to their peers. At a time when federal regulations are forcing both coverage and premium uniformity among Medicare HMOs, this gives Secure Horizons a valuable advantage.

And as an additional gain for PacifiCare, the voluntary turnover among members of the ambassador program has been virtually zero; staff who have been coordinating the program since 1995 can recall no instance of a member disenrolling. One member, who was leaving the area, called to get a list of places where the Secure Horizon plan would be offered so that she would be able to continue in the ambassador program in her new place of residence. Most likely the members who enlist in the ambassador program are more loyal than average to begin with, but their demonstrations of loyalty, as well as the added value they gain by making contributions, tend to raise that loyalty to even higher levels.

Besides the value gained by consumers through the contribution experiences they have, acknowledgment of their contributions adds value to them by enabling them to enjoy a sense of having made a positive difference to an organization they admire, and perhaps to the health of the community as well. This in turn should enhance their self-image and self-esteem, enabling them to feel better about themselves. Coupled with their sense of partnership in a worthy cause, they should gain a sense of belonging to and "owning" a larger endeavor. Further, if acknowledgment is coupled with some form of recognition or reward, they may gain more extrinsic value in addition to these intrinsic benefits.

Contributions to recognize

These can best be selected in light of the direct benefits explicitly promoted and of the indirect benefits logically and credibly connected to those benefits. To gain their greatest sense of sharing in your organization's success and their greatest personal satisfaction, contributing consumers should realize the full scope of their impact, on all of the performance dimensions affected, into the future as well as within the present.

For example, if they have referred five new patients or plan members, the value of their contribution includes the direct volume and revenue effect of that new business. Added value may include a positive influence on employee job security and morale and on quality and efficiency where they are enhanced through increased volume. Since referred customers tend to be more satisfied and loyal than those who are self-referred, ambassador contributions include the greater loyalty and an increased probability of contributions among referred peers.[8]

Acknowledging to consumers the full extent and value of their contributions is not without risk, of course. It opens the possibility that some consumers will feel that they have returned more value to your organization than they received. Any such sense of unfair gains to the parties will undermine the relationship, so you should be both careful to monitor their perceptions on the subject in ongoing evaluations and prepared to promote perceived equity via the sharing step if needed.[9]

Fully identified and evaluated contributions by consumers will be used when recognizing their value internally, and should have been tracked. Any under-recognition of such value when reminding consumers of their contributions carries the chance that they will realize you are keeping "two sets of books" on their value, and will undermine if not destroy their loyalty. It is better to manage the risks involved in their being fully aware of their importance to you than to run the risks of deceiving them.

Wherever consumers have gained personal benefit as part of their contribution experience—whether intrinsic benefits such as learned skills, enjoyment, and socializing, or extrinsic ones such as rewards and incentives—these should be included in reminders. This will add to their overall perceptions of value gained, and could help prevent or counteract the risk that some will feel they have given more than they have gained.

It is important that your acknowledgment to each consumer contributor states precisely the unique value that he or she has contributed and the way in which the individual, or household where applicable, has accomplished it. Because contributions are tracked best on an individual basis, you should have consumer-specific data to use in your acknowledgments, and individualized reminders are far more powerful than general thanks. Moreover, by tying the recognition of particular value contributed to specific consumers and their actions, you are heightening consumers' awareness of which of their actions contributed a particular benefit, thereby promoting more valuable future contributions.

When it comes to managing contributions, think of loyal consumers as human resources in much the same way as employees. They need to know the effects of their actions on specific performance dimensions in order to guide their own decisions regarding those actions.[10] Self-motivated consumers, like employees, can think up their own ways to contribute once they know how their actions make a difference.

Recognition should not be limited to the contributions of the individual consumer. In addition, contributors should get summaries of the contributions and value that their peers have returned to give them a sense of belonging to their peer group of contributors. This added value will further promote their loyalty, and moreover, it will remind them of the perhaps forgotten (or even unknown) potential of other contributory roles and actions for them to consider.

Ways to recognize contributions

Your recognition of consumer contributions involves questions and answers identical to your reminders to them of the benefits they have gained. Any combination of individualized reports, segment summaries, and population-wide summaries may be used, since each serves a different purpose. You can acknowledge significant contributions made by particular acts immediately after they are made and include them later, for double effect, in an "annual report" of the overall contributions made by individuals and households.

One physician made a habit of acknowledging individual loyal patients by recognizing their value on the anniversary of their first visit, and thanking them. Similar acknowledgments on patients' birthdays can work just as well.[11] Health plans, given the importance of reenrollment, can time annual acknowledgments to precede the reenrollment decision period by a week or two, together with reminders of benefits delivered. Combining reminders and acknowledgments in the same package—if not in the same message—makes sense, saving communications costs and promoting the sense of partnership.

Inbound communications, that is, Web sites or other means of access enabling consumers to obtain information on the benefits they have gained and self-evaluation devices letting them figure out on their own what they have gained, are fine for reminding consumers of value gained. When acknowledging their contributions, however, always make the communications outbound. You shouldn't expect consumers to find out for themselves, because many will not, and you will risk sending the wrong message to those who do. If you're aware of someone's help, you should be willing to devote your own resources to acknowledging it and not expect the consumer to find out for him- or herself.

Recognition of consumers can include asking their feelings about their specific contributions and about any benefits they gained thereby: self-esteem, respect by others, sense of accomplishment, sense of making a positive difference, or any others they name. This serves to remind them of the specific benefits they have gained, as it does in the value delivery chain, while it ties such gains directly to their return-value contributions. It should help confirm and reinforce their contribution behavior.

Noncontributors

Reasons to tell others about consumers' contributions

Although loyal contributors are easily the most important and logical group to acknowledge, advantages can be gained through reminding noncontributing consumers who have some kind of relationship with you of the contributions others have made. It will at least promote their consciousness of such contributions—both that you desire them and that their peers have made them—and thereby enhance your contribution promotion efforts.

To some extent it may add some "peer pressure" when these non-contributors learn that large numbers of consumers just like them have contributed value. It will also show your awareness of such contributions and the fact that you appreciate them enough to publicize them. Like all steps in the Loyalty Marketing Wheel, the acknowledgment of contributions to noncontributors may be tested via split treatments to see if it makes enough difference in future contributions to cover the costs of the effort.

Contributions to make known to noncontributors

The contributions to remind noncontributors about should include both the overall pattern and significance of the contributions made by their peers as well as specific examples of individual contributions. Telling them about the difference contributors have made and your appreciation of them should heighten noncontributors' receptivity to the general idea of returning value. Describing specific examples will remind them of what is both desirable and feasible and will enable them to realize that you recognize and acknowledge the importance of individuals.

Approaches for acknowledging contributions to noncontributors

Regular summaries of peer contributions, both the actions and their value to the organization, can be made as part of annual reports or other routine communications to loyal consumers. The timing for such reports need not be specific for individual noncontributors because they will get overall summaries rather than individualized reports. Unless such reports are found to promote reenrollment, they need not be timed for reenrollment decisions. They should be specific to consumers with whom you have a relationship, however, so targeted communications channels such as e-mail or direct mail should be used in preference to mass media.

Internal Stakeholders

Reasons to remind internal stakeholders

Reminding internal stakeholders of the value contributed by loyal consumers should be as much a part of the loyalty marketing process as reminding them of value delivered to consumers. It should help them all—staff, management, board members, partners, and shareholders—to appreciate the importance of consumers and the value of their loyalty.[12] It should also confirm for internal decision makers the reasons for investing in loyalty marketing and reinforce their support for both the overall effort and future contribution promotions.

Reminders to staff of these contributions should also serve to acknowledge staff contributions in achieving consumer loyalty and any staff role played in eliciting particular contributions. This should be part of a systematic "internal marketing" approach to enlist the enthusiastic cooperation and creative investment of staff in the loyalty marketing effort.[13] Reports of the contribution value gained should be coupled for employees with results in performance evaluations and recognition/ reward systems.

The contributions to serve as employee reminders

In reminding employees you should cite the full value, direct and indirect, of consumers' contributions with special emphasis on the benefits of most value to employees. The impact on job security of increased referrals or retention, for example, may be more important to employees than effects on profit. Contributions to quality and to disease management outcomes, for example, may be more important to health professionals, although all employees may gain a sense of pride from quality enhancement. Find out the most important here by testing the comparable effects of contributions on employee morale and loyalty.

Physicians may be interested in learning the ways in which consumer contributions have enhanced their professional and personal lives. Consumers acting as self-care providers or self-managers may have reduced dramatically, for example, the number of interruptions that on-call physicians get. Consumer donations may have made it possible to acquire equipment or improve facilities, benefits always important to physicians.

Managers, executives, and board members may be particularly interested in consumer contributions to annual objectives, strategic aspirations, and problem solutions. Shareholders may focus on profitability and asset value. Although the same overall list and value of consumer contributions may be desired by all of these stakeholder groups, it may prove worthwhile to prepare customized versions of the overall report, emphasizing the contributions most important to each group. Tests can be used to determine if customized reports are more worthwhile to invest in than uniform reports.

As with reports to consumers as a group, include both overall summaries of contributions together with their impact on organizational performance, and individual cases, that is, descriptions of particularly dramatic and heartwarming examples. While a statistical summary may give the most accurate and complete picture of the overall value contributed by loyal consumers, a good anecdote can have far greater and more lasting emotional impact. So use both.

Ways to present contributions as reminders to internal stakeholders

Take advantage of existing, ongoing communications vehicles, such as newsletters, periodic reports, and annual reports. In addition, whenever individual consumer contributions have been particularly dramatic, include case examples in memos, on bulletin boards, and via other vehicles not used for summary reporting. Have employees and managers report on particularly powerful examples in meetings.

In addition to clamping onto existing communications vehicles, create special quarterly or annual summaries of consumer contributions to reinforce ongoing stories and reports. Putting all of the contribution statistics, with discussions and estimates of their total impact on the organization, should help internal stakeholders appreciate the value of consumer loyalty and remind them of the ongoing examples they have seen.

Community Stakeholders

Why tell "outsiders"?

Reporting to the public at large on the nature and extent of contributions made by your loyal consumer patients or plan members should first promote a general public perception of your organization as a good one. The sheer number of loyal consumers you can point to can show the popularity of your organization. The inclusion of measures of contribution value shows how much you appreciate consumers, and should have distinct public relations value. For a beleaguered health plan, the combined reports of overall quality of life benefits to consumers and summaries of consumer reciprocity can go a long way in countering popular "managed care bashing."

Public acknowledgments of consumer contributions can also remind government and other oversight agencies of the degree of public support you enjoy. One of the tests of a charitable, tax-exempt organization, for example, is how much the public has contributed to it, not just how much it has contributed to the community.[14] You can protect any tax-exempt status by reminding regulators of both the benefits you have delivered to the community and the benefits they have contributed in return. And demonstrating clear and significant public support can reinforce the effect of consumers' lobbying efforts and offer some protection against regulatory damage.

Contributions to tell community stakeholders about

Here also, you should use a combination of statistical summaries and case examples, for the same reason it works for internal stakeholders. Particular stakeholders may be interested in particular contributions, so by all means ask them what they'd like to see. Where you can report a trend of increasing contributions, include multiyear data. Choose your intended effect on particular stakeholders and tailor your reports accordingly.

Approaches for reminding community stakeholders

Try a combination of press releases or feature stories, and of overall summaries and high-interest case examples, for ongoing reminders of the contributions consumers are making. These will serve as your own further recognition of contributors and to stimulate noncontributors in addition to reaching internal and external stakeholders. In addition, where particular stakeholder groups or organizations are important enough, prepare separate reports or make special presentations to them. As with all of the loyalty marketing steps, test the value of both the step and the particular approaches to each step for each stakeholder group subject to your investment.

Connections

The recognition step supports the promotion process by reminding consumers of the value they have contributed, and of any they have gained, based on the information you gathered in the monitoring step. Recognition is likely also to initiate or reinforce interest in the idea of sharing by acknowledging to consumers their amount of contribution. Further, it prepares the organization for the sharing process by reminding its stakeholders of the amount that consumers have contributed.

Figure 9-2   Recognition Connections

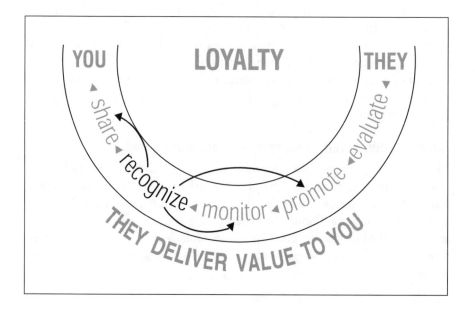

Action Recommendations

✓ Select the consumers whose contributions you intend to acknowledge: they should be everyone who has made a measured, positive contribution. _____

✓ Identify the impact that each individual or group contributor has made to the organization's performance, and estimate the dollar value of that impact. _____

✓ Identify the impact that the contribution experience itself has had on consumers, whether they are more loyal or less, more or less willing to make additional contributions, and so on. Evaluate enough prior to your acknowledgment of their contributions to enable you to pinpoint the difference the acknowledgment makes. _____

✓ Select the form of acknowledgment—for example, public or private, individual or collective—that you will make to contributors and whatever form of recognition you will include, from simple thanks to other forms of appreciation. _____

✓ Decide if you will include some form of sharing with contributors, and design the acknowledgment to complement sharing, if applicable. _____

✓ Inform internal and external stakeholders, as well as noncontributing consumers, of the contributions made by loyal contributors. _____

✓ Prepare for whatever sharing of value contributed you will include. _____

✓ Prepare to evaluate the acknowledgment step in terms of its impact on consumer loyalty. _____

References

1. Beckham, D. 1996. "The Engine of Choice." *Healthcare Forum Journal* 39, no. 4 (July/August): 58–64.

2. Albrecht, K., and L. Bradford. 1990. *The Service Advantage*. Homewood, IL: Dow Jones—Irwin.

3. Bell, C. 1994. *Customers as Partners: Building Relationships That Last*. San Francisco: Berrett-Koehler.

4. Bell, C., and R. Zemke. 1992. *Managing Knock Your Socks Off Service*. New York: AMACOM.

5. Carey, J. 1976. "A Test of Positive Reinforcement of Customers." *Journal of Marketing* 40, no. 4 (October): 98–104.

6. Fisk, T., C. Brown, K. Cannizzaro, and B. Naftal. 1990. "Creating Patient Satisfaction and Loyalty." *Journal of Health Care Marketing* 10, no. 2 (June): 5–15.

7. Edlin, M. 1999. "Outta Sight! Out of Mind." *Managed Healthcare* 9, no. 3 (March): 30–33.

8. Peppers, D., and M. Rogers. 1993. *The One to One Future: Building Relationships One Customer at a Time*. New York: Doubleday.

9. Baron, G. 1997. *Friendship Marketing: Growing Your Business by Cultivating Strategic Relationships*. Grants Pass, OR: Oasis Press.

10. Bowen, D. 1986. "Managing Customers as Human Resources in Service Organizations." *Human Resources Management* (fall): 371–83.

11. Bernstein, A., and D. Freiermuth. 1988. *The Health Professional's Marketing Handbook*. Chicago: Yearbook Medical.

12. Baron, G. 1996. "The Four Stages of a Loyal Business Relationship." *Marketing News* 30, no. 19 (9 September): 7.

13. Starkweather, R., and C. Steinbacher. 1998. "Job Satisfaction Affects the Bottom Line." *HR Magazine* 43, no. 10 (September): 110–12.

14. Hascal, K. 1998. "The Healing Place Helps People Turn Their Lives Around." *Inside Preventive Care* 4, no. 6 (September): 4–6.

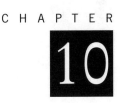

SHARING THE VALUE OF CONTRIBUTIONS

Figure 10-1

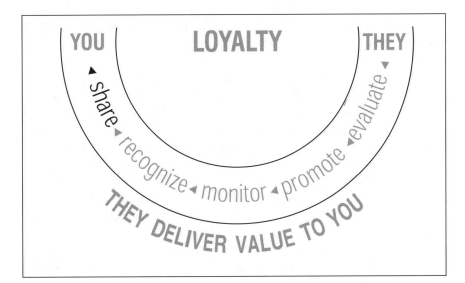

I T MAY seem a revolutionary idea to share with consumers the value they have contributed to your organization. After all, giving back any part of the value contributed automatically reduces the extent to which the contributed value benefits the organization. But such sharing is common practice in most loyalty marketing efforts in other industries, even if it is often not described as a sharing process. And sharing in the value contributed may be among the most powerful ways of promoting consumer loyalty, which, after all, is what this book is all about.

This chapter covers three key questions: *why* you should consider sharing value, *what* value (really how much) to share with consumers, and *how* to share it. Having monitored and recognized the total value, that is, the complete performance benefit impact of consumer contributions, the full potential of the value that can be shared has already been established. While the idea of sharing value with the consumers who contributed it may seem strange at first, by the time you have read the reasons for sharing and the ways to do it, the idea may appear a bit more reasonable.

Benefits of Sharing

Sharing of value contributed with the people who contributed it is a well-established practice in management. Profit sharing with managers has been used by the *Au Bon Pain* chain of retail bakery-restaurants, for example, to significantly improve employee and customer satisfaction and retention.[1] Profit and gain sharing with employees is a common practice in healthcare.[2] Sharing profits with shareholders is virtually essential. Sharing with the community is a well-established practice in healthcare.[3]

Sharing profits with customers is an equally common practice and a significant component of most loyalty marketing programs. Frequent flyer miles and frequent guest awards are ways of sharing in the revenues and profits that highly loyal customers bring to airlines and hotels. Special offers, gifts, and discount coupons do the same with retail store customers.[4] Sharing the gain (and occasionally even the pain) with stakeholders is a way of aligning their incentives with yours, of gaining and maintaining their trust, and of thereby promoting their loyalty.[5]

Sharing with customers the risks and rewards of initiatives and investments is common practice among vendors, even in healthcare. Advertising agencies can share in the results they achieve for providers and plans, for example.[6] Disease management vendors are including the sharing of savings achieved with their managed care clients.[7] One vendor of a computer system developed to prevent medication errors includes a share of the cost savings that result with its hospital and physician clients.[8]

General Electric offers to share risks and rewards with healthcare purchasers of its products; GE advertises that it will help its customers meet cost, productivity, and quality challenges by sharing its expertise and sharing in the results.[9] Alta Bates hospital system shared the savings brought about by its medical staff with the physicians, at the rate of 50 percent of first-year savings, 30 percent of savings for the second year, and 20 percent of its savings in the third year achieved through reengineering efforts.[10]

Although the practice of sharing value gained with *customers* is rare, compared to sharing with internal stakeholders, it is by no means unheard of. Centennial Medical Center in Nashville, Tennessee has included sharing as part of its Business Health Service Division's marketing strategy with employers. It has devoted a one percent share of its gross receipts from each employer client to complimentary wellness programs for each. Its strategy enabled Centennial to increase the number of direct contracting employers from one to 18, and to get into the provider networks of all but one of the dominant MCOs in the market, as compared to fewer than half of them before embarking on the strategy.[11]

The basic underlying concept is that sharing value with consumers, as with any other stakeholder group, can bring them closer to the organization in terms of loyalty and shared interests, and can help in promoting the particular actions through which they have contributed that value. As Bell put it, "People will care, if they share." And if they perceive that they somehow are sharing in the value they contribute, they are likely to feel more like your partner, more a member of the family than a guest or a stranger.[12]

You may recall that with the growing popularity of one:one marketing and its focus on consumers have led Peppers and Rogers to suggest a unique relationship proposition for the new marketing: "The more the customer does on the firm's behalf, the more the firm does on the customer's behalf."[13] Although this proposition could be treated narrowly, focusing only on consumers in their customer role, it clearly encompasses application to all their roles as long as they contribute to "the firm's behalf."

The sharing of the value of contributions with consumer contributors fits particularly well with the empowerment approach to promoting return-value contributions as described in chapter 7. Although gaining agreement on the performance value outcomes to be achieved affects both motivation and guidance, giving empowered consumers the expectation that they will somehow share in the value contributed may greatly add to their motivation. Sharing makes common goals of the outcomes to be achieved, strengthening the sense of partnership desired in loyalty marketing.

When consumers share in the value they contribute, they are less likely to view their relationship with your organization as inequitable in terms of one party gaining more from it. In instances where you have gained significant value from consumers and have tracked and acknowledged that value to them, their awareness may very well lead them to expect some form of sharing. Thus, if you do not share value with them in some way, you may be undermining the loyalty marketing impact of the entire value return chain. If you are trying to create among consumers the perception of partnership, of common goals and values, sharing may be essential: partners share, after all.

What better way to demonstrate that "we're in this together" than to share the results of your partnership with consumers who clearly have contributed to your success; what better way to "walk the talk" of your communications campaigns aimed at creating and strengthening consumer loyalty. With incentives alignment so popular in relations between hospitals and physicians, and between health plans and providers, why not align incentives with consumers? And because you have demonstrably gained from their contributions, you can, after all, afford some sharing. Moreover, if consumers who have made significant contributions see the result only as increased profits for the organization, higher dividends and stock prices for owners, and more outrageous compensation for executives, their motivation to contribute may well disappear.

Risks of Sharing

Sharing the value contributed by consumers is not without its costs and risks, however. Whenever consumers gain personally from their contributions to your mission, success, and survival, their intrinsic sense of well-being and self-worth that accompanies a contribution may be undermined, even wiped out by the extrinsic reward.[14] If patients are rewarded through sharing in the "profits" gained from each patient they refer, for example, they might interpret that reward as a kind of "bribe," and may feel that they are no longer objectively helping their friends and neighbors but have been manipulated into somehow betraying them.[12]

This is especially true when specific methods of sharing value personally with consumers are promised or decided up front. Consumers who have been promised a "finder's fee" for referring a new patient or plan member (my dentist promises a free dinner for two, for example) essentially become independent contractors working for the organization and are no longer disinterested advisors or referral sources for their peers. Even rewarding after the fact, with no enticement beforehand, can have the same effect on subsequent contributions.

The extent of this negative effect may be mitigated by the particular contribution involved, however. A consumer who gets a promised financial reward for a suggestion that saves the organization money or improves its quality may not feel sullied by the reward. It is more likely that the *promise,* later followed by delivery of the personal financial reward, will simply drive out intrinsic motivation. Although a single unpromised (but delivered) reward can have the same effect in weakening intrinsic motivation for subsequent contributions, the effect may be less. Repeated rewards tend to have less impact than that experienced with the first pleasant surprise. And if rewards are not repeated, the influence of extrinsic motivation on eliciting repeated contributions disappears.[15]

Incentives are generally held to be powerful and significant for the short term: to elicit a particular behavior, for instance, such as using an enclosed dollar bill to pre-reward consumers for returning a questionnaire. The trouble is, it is also generally held to be less helpful, and often ineffective, for eliciting repeated or continued behaviors. Monetary rewards have been found to be far less effective, for example, than the intrinsic benefits of the job in motivating employees.[16] Why should they be expected to work with consumers?

Although it may be true, as LeBoeuf claims, that "what gets rewarded gets repeated,"[17] it does not follow that financial incentives are the best rewards, particularly for the long term. Intrinsic rewards, the psychosocial benefits of making a difference, gaining useful knowledge and skills, and enjoying the camaraderie of peers, for example, tend to have far greater lasting power and fewer risks. Extrinsic rewards do not empower people; they create dependency on the rewards, possibly make people feel manipulated, and focus attention on the precise action that will be rewarded—perhaps at the expense of other activities that would prove more advantageous to the organization.[18]

Sharing in the form of personal financial rewards may tempt some consumers to report contributions they never made, compromising self-tracking, survey tracking, and themselves. In many cases, extrinsic incentives affect only people who are already motivated to do what will be rewarded and add little to the probability of their contribution. And once given, the extrinsic reward may so diminish intrinsic motivation that it requires repeated, often increased incentives to motivate repetition. Extrinsic rewards tend to diminish, if not destroy, sincere commitments to the organization and leave only a commitment to getting the reward.[13]

This is not to suggest that personal rewards, particularly financial ones, should never be used as means of sharing with consumers the value they have contributed. It well may be that for some one-time contributions of a particular type, they can work well. They have worked in a wide range of commercial applications, in getting women to initiate prenatal care earlier, or in enticing smokers to attend smoking cessation classes or sedentary consumers to try exercising. It is mainly in the long run that they tend to show their limitations and negative side effects.

A second risk is that employees and other internal stakeholders may feel that they have a right to share in demonstrated gains as well, and may see consumers as rivals for sharing. If you are already sharing performance gains or profits with employees, they may see any sharing with consumers as frivolous and unfair, costing them shares they deserve for their own contributions. Shareholders in particular may object to sharing by noninvestors in any financial way, since that would reduce dividends and undermine share value.

Even external stakeholders may object to the idea of sharing value with your consumer patients or members, particularly if yours is a not-for-profit organization dedicated to serving the community as a whole. They may prefer that you share your gains with everyone in the community rather than only with those patients or members who have made tracked contributions.

To defuse or at least reduce negative reactions by internal stakeholders, it is first essential that they understand that the value added by loyal consumer contributions is new, representing marginal value that would not have been realized otherwise. Thus reporting to internal stakeholders the value contributed by loyal consumers, as described in the recognition step, is crucial to preparing those stakeholders for the idea of sharing. Once they appreciate that no added value would exist to share were it not for consumer contributions, they should be less opposed to the idea of sharing it with them.

Moreover, sharing does not necessarily mean a 50/50 split between the consumer contributors and the organization: it means only a split that consumers will see as fair and motivating. In my experience, when consumers have been asked to describe a fair share or to help in deciding how to spend the added value, they have tended to be conservative rather than greedy. However, where gainsharing with employees or physicians and where dividends to shareholders are clearly committed, these stakeholders have not, in my experience at least, recognized that many others deserve to share.

For external stakeholders, objections to sharing value with consumers should be somewhat mitigated by the fact that consumers are members of the community. Moreover, the sharing of value may well be in the form of community health and other betterment investments. In cases where consumers support, even prefer, the idea of sharing with the community, bringing their own interests into line with community needs and the organization's mission values, the risk of conflict over the sharing of value with external stakeholders greatly decreases. At the same time, the risks that an extrinsic reward will drive out intrinsic motivation and will undermine loyalty virtually disappear when the sharing of value contributed by consumers is in the form of investing for community good and is not of direct personal benefit to any selfish consumer interests.

And, *mirabile dictu,* when value sharing focuses on community benefit, the risk of conflict with internal stakeholders can also diminish. Those of us who have chosen careers in healthcare are almost all driven at least partly by a desire to make a positive difference in our communities.[19] When added value provides the opportunity for the organization to contribute significantly to community health and welfare, most employees, at least in my experience, support the idea. To promote internal acceptance, it is a good idea to reach agreement on the principal, and if possible, the specific applications of sharing, before it becomes imminent, when no real value is there for employees to "lose," rather than either to decide unilaterally on sharing that value or to wait until after it is realized to broach the subject.

Shareholders may be the most reluctant to reduce their personal benefit by sharing some portion of value added by consumers with those consumers. And executives, managers, and employees or physicians who see themselves as losing personal financial gains may be unswayed by plans to reinvest returned value in the community. In such cases, the public relations and long-term reputation impact plus the market impact of community investments—or even the loyalty and long-term financial impact of sharing with consumers—may suffice to show that such sharing is in the personal, even selfish interests of internal stakeholders.

Because the idea of sharing the value contributed by consumers with those consumers is pretty much an untried effort, no way exists to argue for its sure success or to define the best approach for defusing internal or external stakeholder opposition. As with each of the other loyalty marketing steps, trial and evaluation (nobody should assume that errors are necessary) form the best way to test the benefit of the sharing step as well as the efficiency and effectiveness of particular approaches to sharing.

Carrying Out the Sharing Step

Perhaps in no other loyalty marketing step is the question of carrying it out more critical to its success or even to its internal acceptance as an idea. In the best of circumstances, sharing needs preparation. Involvement of the internal stakeholders, and perhaps the external ones as well, in jointly planning the loyalty marketing effort can enable them to see the long-range purposes and expectations of the effort and will help prepare them for sharing. Citing examples of its successful use by other industries may also help stakeholders to picture the long-range benefits of sharing as well as the immediate personal costs to them.

Establishing the Value to Share

The amount of value to be shared, the way in which the value contributed by consumers is shared, *and the decision making required for such sharing* will greatly influence acceptance of the idea by stakeholders as well as the type and amount of effect that sharing has on the loyalty of consumers. The consumers who are to share in value they contribute should be as involved as possible in deciding the amount that will be shared. For contributions that are reflected in clear and direct dollar terms, that is, in increased revenue and reduced costs, your tracking should already have established the amount.

For contributions reflected in other performance dimensions, such as quality, relationships, reputation, or mission achievements, it is more problematic to establish a dollar estimate as a basis for decisions on sharing. As with your own internal estimate of value delivered, described in the monitoring step (chapter 8), a Delphi approach is frequently the best choice for this task. Since the intent is to help in deciding the amount to share with consumers, it makes sense to invite consumers to participate in the Delphi process.

I have used the Delphi process for this purpose by using the kind of report of total value contributed developed in the recognition step (chapter 9) for mass distribution as the basis for the Delphi estimate. Using such a report, you ask consumers to examine the list of total nonfinancial value contributed and to make their best estimate of its worth in dollar terms. Your own experts and staff will also be participants and can supply facts and opinions to help. The consensus estimate reached on total value can be used as the starting point.

The same process can be used to decide on the portion of contributed value to be shared with contributors. The same consumers or a different group of them may be invited to participate. The numbers of participants in each group may be as large or small as you wish, but you should recognize that only those who participate will gain the benefits and bestow the imprimatur of their participation on the decision. In situations where consumer estimates of value or preference for sharing may appear to be unaffordably high, you may keep the number small until you get a better feeling for the result and more comfort in the whole idea.

Spending the Share

Once the estimate of total value and a decision on the total to be shared have been made, a consumer participation approach should be used in deciding how to spend the share.[20] This may include any mix of making up-front suggestions, participating in actual decision processes, and offering feedback on specific proposals. Sharing power with consumers in making such decisions will reinforce the sense of partnership, in addition to delivering the specific benefit of decision-making power.

One item in the loyalty evaluation step, as discussed in chapter 6, should be an investigation into the types and levels of sharing preferred by the consumers from whom you want to elicit contributions of value. As with internal stakeholders, discussing the sharing methods and gaining agreement before any value is established, may prove easier than doing so after the fact. And certainly, including consumers in decisions will work better than will unilateral decisions on your part.

Including consumers in deciding how to share the value they contribute will, first of all, enhance their perceptions of your sense of fairness and of your recognition of their importance and value to your organization. Your contacts with them that arise from their participation in the decision-making effort can (assuming the contacts are not onerous) increase the numbers of experiences you have with each other, enhancing familiarity and promoting their loyalty.

Moreover, where consumers choose a form of sharing that involves an investment in community health and the organization's mission as opposed to personal gains (and this has been the case in the majority of cases in which I've been involved), those consumers gain the added benefit of feeling they are contributing to something worthwhile, something that they can be proud of and that their neighbors will praise them for. Thus the process of being involved in deciding can add significant, loyalty-enhancing benefit to consumers, in addition to promoting their acceptance of the sharing decision itself.

Describing the motivation behind the sharing activity, as well as its actual object and process, may also make a difference in its effect on consumers, and thereby on their perception of the organization and on their long-term loyalty. If rewards are described, when promised and when given, as explicit means of thanking consumers and sharing the benefits with them rather than as the kinds of rewards that are perceived more as bribes, perhaps their negative impact will be less and their positive impact more.

Consider the physician who, as mentioned earlier, offers the free week in his condo to the winner of an annual drawing for all patients who have referred new patients.[21] If that physician describes the reward as his way of enabling his patients to share in his financial success because they have shared in its achievement, perhaps these patients will feel better about being "paid" to refer their friends. If the physician prepares such patients by thanking them and describing how he has been able to help the friends they referred, they will be less likely to suspect untoward manipulation.

Making the shared personal reward a surprise special gift after the fact may be less damaging than promising it before the fact or making the reward a regular feature. Sharing value through a celebration of consumers in general who have contributed value—an annual dinner with entertainment, for example—may be seen as a reasonable way to recognize and reward contributors. Using the value contributed to add to intrinsic benefits for the contributing consumers—such as increasing skills training or hosting more socialization opportunities—may also prove effective.

Community Investment

Perhaps the safest, and in many ways the most powerful, approach to sharing the value contributed is to do so at the community level rather than the personal level. For example, your organization might donate some significant share of financial gains attributed to consumer contributions to a worthy cause in which they have indicated an interest. They may have chosen this cause through participating in the decision process. Because they already know the amount of their contribution to the value you share, thanks to your monitoring and acknowledgment steps, they will gain the sense of having made part of the donation themselves. You should easily be able to ensure that they get a personalized acknowledgment from the cause to which the donation is made, so that they gain further recognition benefit.

You might use the value of their contributions in the "tithing" that many health organizations are doing, donating 10 percent of operating margin to multiple worthy causes in the community.[22] This may prove more popular among consumers than contributing to a single cause. Here, also, they may help decide which causes to contribute to, thereby gaining additional benefit themselves. Moreover, in many cases, these donations can be made in the form of grants for particular programs, so that consumers can feel a part of specific new initiatives as opposed solely to support for the general good. For example, if donations were made for a new neighborhood clinic, each consumer who contributed can feel a part in having built it.

Yet a third approach to sharing contributed value at the community level would be investing in your own mission-focused activities: initiating or expanding health promotion, prevention, early detection, phone counseling and information services, consumer health libraries, prenatal care for uninsured mothers, and any other of your mission causes. As with the preceding approaches, consumers can participate in deciding the particular initiatives to support, thus gaining a greater sense of partnership with you. Finally, knowing that they are "investing" in such programs may motivate them to volunteer or help recruit participants in "their" programs.

By including a consumer vote in your choice of programs to benefit from their share in the value they contribute, you may find that you add significant motivation to consumers to make the contributions that will make the sharing possible.[23] When you are dealing with a sufficiently large value amount, particularly when the value has translated directly or via a Delphi estimate into dollar terms, you may choose to create a foundation or at least a formal body to make such decisions on a regular basis. Including consumers as official members of this body should naturally follow.

When you use a community-focused sharing approach, be sure to clarify to consumers that it is their contributions and the value they have added to the organization's performance that made possible the particular investment selected. This will help them connect their actions both to a positive impact on your organization and to the resulting benefit to the community. They can then feel proud not only of their own contributions, but of your organization, for having chosen to devote resources to the community good.

Your organization, in turn, gains the public relations impact of making contributions to the welfare and quality of life of the community. This should enhance staff and other stakeholder morale, foster pride in your loyal consumer/customers in being associated with you, and make prospects who are considering provider and plan choices more likely to choose you.[24]

To fully mine this form of sharing, make sure that any causes, projects, and mission initiatives to which you donate shares of consumer contributions carefully track and evaluate the beneficial results they are having on the community's health and welfare. Then you should report this impact to contributing consumers as further acknowledgment of the value they have contributed. This gives you yet another loyalty-promoting contact with them. In addition, you can send the same report to noncontributing consumers, to awaken their interest, and to internal and external stakeholders as part of your overall stakeholder relations strategy.

As with all of the loyalty marketing steps and their approaches, all facets of the value-added sharing step can be tested via trial and evaluation; they need not be blindly followed. Given so little experience in the sharing of contributed value, either by itself or as an integral component of the loyalty marketing strategy, some degree of prudence is recommended. On the other hand, based on admittedly limited experience, this particular step has perhaps the greatest potential for the widest impact on the organization and the community it serves. Others have found that investments in the community are well correlated with the organization's own financial performance.[25]

Connections

The sharing of value contributed to your organization by consumers can have a positive effect on the promotion of such contributions, either when promised up front or when used as a recognition and reward for contributors. As consumers gain personal value, or the sense of contributing to the community through sharing, the value return chain itself becomes a self-reinforcing loop, as the value that is shared confirms and re-motivates consumers to at least consider repeating or adding contributions. Sharing turns the value return chain into a value delivery chain for consumers who contribute or might do so.

Sharing in itself also serves as a powerful form of recognition. As the sharing of value is reported to contributors, other loyal consumers, and the general public, the contributors are gaining an additional form of recognition, reminding them of the impact their contributions have had on community health or other worthy causes. More important, it creates or reinforces the sense of partnership both in making contributions and in being a loyal consumer. It paves the way for the next rotation of the Loyalty Marketing Wheel.

Figure 10-2   Sharing Connections

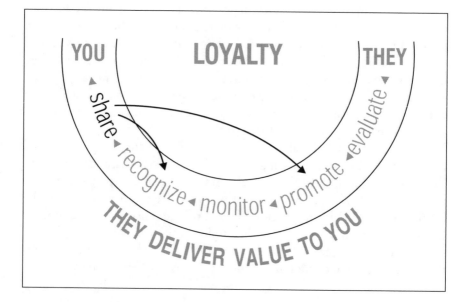

Action Recommendations

✓ Identify the purposes you expect or hope to serve through sharing value with contributors. _____

✓ Decide whether to include value sharing in your loyalty marketing strategy and in any particular contribution solicitation effort. _____

✓ Examine the dollar value of contributions made and select an approach to deciding on ways to share it, with particular attention to identifying those who will be included in the decision: the internal and external stakeholders and the consumer contributors themselves. _____

✓ Select the best approach to sharing, on an individual contributor, on a collective, or on a community basis: note the risk—that individual rewards may drive out the intrinsic contributor rewards, making consumers dependent on future extrinsic rewards. _____

✓ Track the impact of value sharing on its recipients: the difference it is making to contributors or the community. _____

✓ Report to all interested parties, internal and external stakeholders and both contributor and noncontributor consumers, the methods you used to share value and the impact the sharing-distribution had. _____

✓ Prepare to evaluate the effect of sharing, including control versus experimental comparisons where you shared and did not share, and split-test the different approaches to sharing. _____

References

1. Heskett, J., E. Sasser, and L. Schlesinger. 1997. *The Service Profit Chain.* New York: Free Press.
2. "Kaiser Ties Nurses' Bonus to Bottom Line." *Business & Health* 14, no. 3 (March 1996): 9.
3. Pittman, M., D. Bohr, and B. Rosman. 1998. "Invest in Tomorrow: Healthcare Tithing." *Healthcare Forum Journal* 41, no. 4 (July/August): 36–38.
4. Srinivasan, M. 1996. "When It Comes to Loyal Customers, the I's Have It." *Marketing News* 30, no. 14 (1 July): 4.
5. Whitney, J. 1994. *The Trust Factor.* New York: McGraw-Hill.
6. Kelly, T., and P. Kelly. 1998. "Agency-Client Relationships: Putting Both Parties at Risk for Performance." Alliance for Healthcare Strategy and Marketing Advertising Conference, 8 June.
7. Burns, J. 1997. "DM Vendors Talk the Talk and Walk the Walk—And They Guarantee Their Results." *Managed Healthcare* 7, no. 8 (August): 18–21, 25.
8. Bridge Medical. 1998. Promotional materials, San Diego, CA.
9. "Sharing to Gain: Why and How Providers and Suppliers Should Cooperate for the Future." Advertisement in *Health Systems Review* 28, no. 2 (March/April 1995): 12–13.

10. Weber, D. 1998. "Alta Bates Uses Its Own Doctors as Reengineering Consultants for a Share in the Savings that Result from Redesign Initiatives." *Strategies for Healthcare Excellence* (January): 1–6.

11. "A Hospital Makes Business Its Business." *Profiles in Healthcare Marketing* no. 48 (July/August 1992): 2–13.

12. Bell, C. 1994. *Customers as Partners: Building Relationships that Last,* p. 132, pp. 70–81. San Francisco: Berrett-Koehler.

13. Peppers, D., and M. Rogers. 1993. *The One to One Future: Building Relationships One Customer at a Time,* p. 62. New York: Doubleday.

14. Kohn, A. 1993. "Why Incentives Cannot Work." *Harvard Business Review* 71, no. 5 (September/October): 54–63.

15. Chapman, L. 1998. "The Role of Incentives in Health Promotion." *The Art of Health Promotion* 2, no. 3 (July/August): 1–8.

16. Herzberg, F. 1968. "One More Time: How DO You Motivate Employees?" *Harvard Business Review* 46, no. 1 (January/February).

17. LeBoeuf, M. 1985. *The Greatest Management Principle in the World.* New York: Berkeley Books.

18. Argyris, C. 1998. "Empowerment: The Emperor's New Clothes." *Harvard Business Review* 76, no. 3 (May/June): 98–105.

19. Friedman, E. 1998. "What Business Did You Say We Were In?" *Healthcare Forum Journal* 41, no. 4 (July/August): 8–12.

20. Miller, J. 1993. *The Corporate Coach: How to Build a Team of Loyal Customers and Happy Employees.* New York: St. Martin's Press.

21. "Fun & Games Create Big Profits." *The Practice Builder* 11, no. 7 (July 1993): 1–2.

22. DeWolf, L., and B. Giloth. 1998. "Strategies for Outcomes Measurement." *Healthcare Forum Journal* 41, no. 4 (July/August): 32–34.

23. Smith, S., and D. Alcorn. 1991. "Cause Marketing: A New Direction in the Marketing of Corporate Responsibility." *Journal of Services Marketing* 5, no. 4 (fall): 21–37.

24. Gaines, C. 1998. "Next Step in Cause Marketing: Businesses Start Own Nonprofits." *Marketing News* 32, no. 21 (12 October): 4.

25. Waddock, S., and S. Graves. 1997. "The Corporate Social Performance—Financial Performance Link." *Strategic Management Journal* 32 (2): 303–19.

EPILOGUE: STARTING OVER

ONE OF the reasons why the loyalty marketing chains have been presented in this "wheel" metaphor is that they are intended to rotate through the same steps over and over again, moving the wheel. The Loyalty Marketing Wheel reflects the new challenge that loyalty marketing presents to health plans and providers: to be loyal to consumers in order to achieve and retain their loyalty. When we recognize how "few consumers perceive a planned [healthcare] system that operates on their behalf . . . [rather one that is] seen as designed to block access, reduce quality and limit spending, all at the expense of patients," we are faced with a serious handicap in this regard.[1]

Completing the Loop

Essentially, our challenge is to demonstrate to consumers that we value our relationships with them and theirs with us, not merely for their contributions to our performance, significant though they may be, but because we value them as persons. We are challenged to prove that we value people as ends in themselves, rather than as means to our own ends.[2] We face a kind of Catch-22 here. Unless we appreciate consumers as ends in themselves, we risk never achieving the potential: their contributing to our ends—but if we try too hard with consumers to achieve our ends, we risk not appreciating them or being perceived not to appreciate them as ends in themselves.

We can show consumers, in any number of ways, that we trust and value them, for example, beyond achieving their trust in and valuation of us.

Offering loyal consumers special access to the organization's executives, in addition to normal customer service lines, has worked for years in business-to-business marketing. Giving consumers some control over the relationship and the decisions made in the pursuit and mining of loyalty both demonstrates the organization's trust of them and promotes their trust in the organization.[3]

You demonstrate your loyalty to consumers when you avoid engaging in behaviors that exploit them for the organization's self-interests and that damage their interests. Protecting patients' privacy and confidentiality is a clear, essential demonstration of respect for consumers. Selling information about them without their permission and not for their benefit can be an early loyalty destroyer. Misleading consumers in order to gain particular contributions, as reported about one pharmaceutical firm when it promoted lobbying efforts by its customers, would be equally destructive.[4]

The Golden Rule is one guide to keeping the organization on target for showing its own loyalty to consumers, but so is the modest variation on the theme: "Do Unto Others As They Would Have Themselves Done To."[5] Do not apply your own values and assume that they reflect your consumers' wishes. Show your commitment to them by going the extra mile in serving them, by demonstrating your trust in them, and by including at least occasional proactive and pleasant surprises based on your knowledge of them as individuals. Be willing to start first, to model the kind of loyal relationship you want by being loyal first.[6]

Ensure that your organization and its stakeholders begin the loyalty marketing effort with a sense of "abundance".[7] This means, first, being confident enough in the organization's resources, purposes, and probability of success to invest in the effort up front for an extended period before realizing any payoff; and in not expecting a return on investment in the same quarter or year that the investment is made. It also requires stakeholder willingness, on a consistent and equitable basis, to promise a share of, or at least to share with consumers after the fact, the value they contribute.

Loyalty marketing requires organizations to shift to a longer-term horizon. This includes making long-term investments for a long-term payoff.[8] It also means shifting the marketing horizon from "during" to durable benefits, to consumers' gains from long-term relationships with your organization, rather than the benefits received only during encounters and other transactions. Most of all, it requires an extension of vision beyond the structure and process features, events, and attributes—even beyond clinical outcomes—that occupy so much marketing attention, to the quality of life benefits and costs that plans and providers can and do deliver to consumers.

The essential focus of the Loyalty Marketing Wheel is most importantly on the value that health plans and providers can deliver to consumers, through transactions and relationships. The revenue and profit that result from customer transactions and relationships, and even the contributions of value that consumers make as expressions of their loyalty, are best viewed as the rewards for delivering value, *not* the objective of loyalty marketing.[9]

The more consumers we can bring to the "champion" or "advocate" level of loyalty, the more likely we can gain dramatic benefit from them. As we increasingly identify shared values with them and align intrinsic benefits rather than relying on extrinsic incentives, we become more likely to achieve and maintain those levels of loyalty.[10] The more we empower consumers to contribute their types and amounts of actual and potential value, the more we become empowered ourselves to gain both personal and professional satisfaction as well as organizational success.

If we view consumers as means to our own ends, rather than as ends in themselves, however, that is sure to corrupt our thinking and behavior and to destroy, or at least drastically reduce, our potential for achieving loyalty and realizing its full value. The exploitation of consumer loyalty for selfish gains is simply not a practical strategy in the long run; consumers will catch on. Loyalty marketing requires a careful balance between striving for loyalty for its own sake, and promoting returns of value by consumers who are loyal. The two are not incompatible, but they require a continuous balancing of interests.

With such balance, and with careful and consistent use of the Loyalty Marketing Wheel's basic logic and constituent steps, health plans and providers can gain significant competitive advantage. This may come from focusing on relationships while rivals focus only on transactions— on delivering value while rivals focus only on gaining it for themselves, on envisioning longer-term horizons while rivals insist on a short-term payoff—or from focusing on value while rivals deal only with structure and process. Any of these distinctions may make loyalty marketing advantageous both strategically and tactically. The combination of any or all of these distinctions will increase the advantage that much more.

Once you appreciate the full potential value of consumers, as loyal plan members and patients, you may see some parallels with the potential value of employees, partners, and other stakeholders traditionally thought closer and more important to the organization. With this realization should come a willingness to examine, adapt, and apply your knowledge of other loyal stakeholders to the pursuit of consumer loyalty. Virtually all of the concepts and techniques useful in creating loyalty among any categories of people should prove applicable to consumers, and vice versa.

When you start over, the learning step in the value delivery chain also becomes an evaluation step relative to the value return chain and the Loyalty Marketing Wheel as a whole. You will want to check on the total value returned to the organization from promoting, monitoring, recognizing, and sharing value returns: how have these steps affected your performance, particularly your relationships? You should also check the separately added value of each step in the value return chain and the ways in which each step added its value as well as all approaches to each step when you tested more than one.

In this way the learning step, when repeated, becomes the basis for deciding on the success of the overall strategy of loyalty marketing and on the effectiveness of the methods the organization used. It also serves as the start for repetitions of the management, promising, tracking, and reminding steps in the next round of marketing, whether aimed at new and better transactions or at particular return value contributions. The repeated motion of the wheel should be even more successful, thanks to the lessons learned in the evaluation step and in the repeated learning step.

The value delivery chain and the value return chain operate independently, although they are logically connected as a wheel or reinforcing loop. You may have to deliver value many times to some consumers before they reach the stage of returning any value beyond that of a continuing customer. Or you may find that some consumers repeatedly return value to you after you have delivered significant value only once. Although the wheel functions as a realistic model for your relations with a population, the separate chains may reflect better your ongoing relationship with particular individuals.

The more you customize your loyalty marketing efforts, the more you will employ separately the delivery and the return chains. The frequency of your opportunities to deliver value to individuals will depend on a variety of only semi-predictable and partially manageable factors, including the incidence of disease and injury and the interests of consumers in health promotion, prevention, self-care, and disease management. Loyalty marketing combines proactive with reactive initiatives and population-focused with individual-focused activities.

The references provided in this book, particularly those books listed at the end of this chapter, are recommended as further reading for additional insights into the potential value of consumer loyalty and for additional suggestions on achieving it. Consumer loyalty represents a new challenge, and those health plans and providers who take it on will be pioneers, adding to our knowledge of loyalty marketing in healthcare and adding,

Figure E-1 New Roles for Research

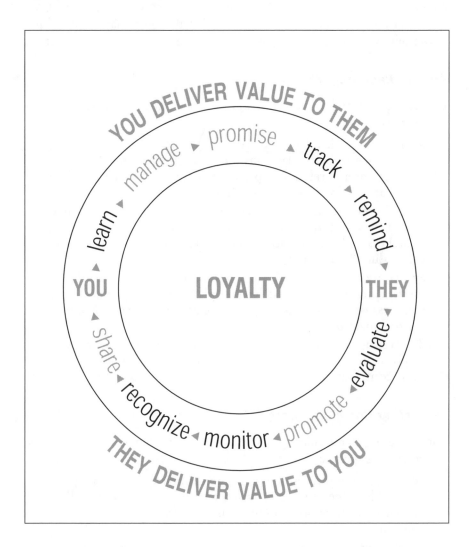

as well, to the quality of life of patients and plan members and to the quality of the community and the health services organization.

New Tasks for Marketers and Managers

The Loyalty Marketing Wheel includes a number of new tasks for marketing specialists and for managers. All of these tasks require not new skills but new applications for current skills—new ways of using the techniques of traditional transaction-focused marketing—for relationship purposes.

These new tasks will challenge marketers to allocate their time and resources and to increase such resources through the support of their organizations for the new tasks. They will challenge managers to rethink both their own roles and the roles and resources they assign to marketers.

Market Researchers

For market researchers, the tasks are those of applying research techniques to:

- learning about loyalty by discovering the factors that make a difference to particular consumers when they choose both transactions and relationships, and when they decide to stick with one relationship rather than to shop for another;
- learning the extent to which consumers perceive that they have gained the value promised, expected, and desired; their level of awareness and appreciation of such value; and their attribution of such value to its source;
- evaluating the status of loyalty among consumers after the implementation of value delivery and the state of preparation and readiness of loyal consumers to make return value contributions to the organization; and
- discovering the kinds of appeals most likely to produce a positive response in loyal consumers: the desired type and amount or return value contributions.

Marketing Communicators

For marketing communicators, whether in advertising or public relations, the challenges include:

- devising and implementing communications that not only promise irresistible value but are consistent with the value that will be delivered, thus promoting loyalty as well as recruitment of consumers;
- developing communications that remind consumers of value they have gained, that promote their awareness and appreciation of such value, that foster their attribution of such value to the organization—and that remind other stakeholders of the same delivered value;
- implementing communications that promote return value contributions as effectively as the communications that attract consumers to the organization's products and services; and
- employing communications that remind consumers, individually and collectively, of the value they have contributed to the organization,

Figure E-2   New Roles for Communications

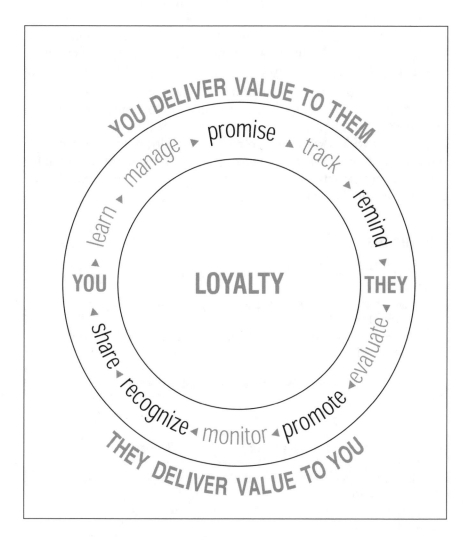

and making consumers and other stakeholders aware of the ways in which the organization is sharing that value.

Managers

Managers in pursuit of consumer loyalty will also have some new tasks:

- managing the entire loyalty marketing effort, strategy, tactics, and resource allocations to promote effective and efficient achievement of loyalty goals and objectives;

- managing the delivery of value for continuous improvement of the organization's success in improving the quality and quantity of life of consumers; and
- devising an approach to sharing that meets the needs and expectations of consumers and of internal and external stakeholders.

The Loyalty Marketing Wheel is intended to help marketers and managers carry out their present roles and new challenges in ways that consciously recognize both their importance and their interdependence. Loyalty marketing holds enormous promise for healthcare organizations, plans, and providers who can apply it successfully, both for themselves and for consumers. It is by recognizing and addressing the potential for delivering and gaining value, and their inseparable connection, that we can all gain from loyalty marketing.

References

1. Adamson, G. 1998. "In Your Face." *Managed Healthcare* 8, no. 4 (April): 15–16, 21–22.
2. Chappel, T. 1993. *The Soul of a Business: Managing for Profit and the Common Good.* New York: Bantam Books.
3. Fournier, S., S. Dobscha, and D. G. Mick. 1998. "Preventing the Premature Death of Relationship Marketing." *Harvard Business Review* 76, no. 1 (January/February): 42–51.
4. Drinkard, J. 1997. "Drug Company Accused of Misleading Asthmatics." *Denver Post* (22 August): 9A.
5. Albrecht, K., and L. Bradford. 1990. *The Service Advantage.* Homewood, IL: Dow Jones–Irwin.
6. Baron, G. 1997. *Friendship Marketing: Growing Your Business by Cultivating Strategic Relationships.* Grants Pass, OR: Oasis Press.
7. Bell, C. 1994. *Customers as Partners: Building Relationships That Last.* San Francisco: Berrett-Koehler.
8. Peltier, J. 1998. "Relationship Building: Measuring Service Quality Across Health Care Encounters." *Marketing Health Services* 18, no. 3 (fall): 17–24.
9. Reichheld, F. 1996. "Introduction" In *The Quest for Loyalty,* edited by F. Reichheld, pp. xv–xxvi. Boston: Harvard Business School.
10. Cross, R., and J. Smith. 1995. *Customer Bonding: 5 Steps to Lasting Customer Loyalty.* Lincolnwood, IL: NTC Business Books.

About the Author

R. Scott MacStravic, Ph.D. is principal of the consulting firm Demand Engineering in Golden, Colorado, and teaches health services marketing at the University of Colorado, Denver. Before going into business for himself, he was Vice President for Marketing and Strategy at Provenant Health Partners in Denver, a multihospital system now part of Centura Health and Catholic Health Initiatives. Prior to joining Provenant in 1989 he was Vice President for Planning and Marketing at Health and Hospital Services, Inc., now PeaceHealth in Bellevue, Washington. He has also taught at the Medical College of Virginia, the University of Washington, and the University of Southern California.

Dr. MacStravic earned his Ph.D. in hospital administration at the University of Minnesota and his undergraduate degree at Harvard University. He is a member of the Alliance for Healthcare Strategy and Marketing and is on the editorial boards of the journals *Health Care Strategic Management* and *Strategic Health Care Marketing*. He is the author of ten books and more than 180 articles on healthcare strategy and marketing.